I0094362

Protect Yourself:

From Ebola to Zika and
From MRSA to Hospital Acquired Infections:
How to Avoid Contagious Diseases

Brent W. Laartz, MD FIDSA

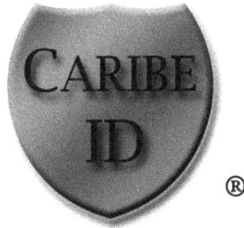

Publisher Caribe ID, LLC

Copyright © 2016 by Brent W. Laartz, MD FIDSA and Caribe ID, LLC.

Cover Art and Design by Jessica Pecoraro

Proofing and Editing by John Toney, MD and Sarah DiMonaco

All rights reserved. No part of this work may be reproduced or transmitted in any form or by any means, electronic or mechanical, including photocopying, recording, or by any information storage or retrieval system, without the prior written permission of the copyright owner and the publisher.

ISBN-13: 978-0-9982054-1-0 (Paperback), 978-0-9982054-0-3 (Ebook)

Publisher: Caribe ID, LLC

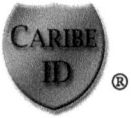

For information on distribution, translations, or bulk sales, please contact Caribe ID, LLC directly:

Caribe ID, LLC
1840 Mease Drive, Suite 319
Safety Harbor, FL 34695

Library of Congress Control Number 2016918237

Laartz, Brent W

Protect Yourself: From Ebola to Zika and From MRSA to Hospital Acquired Infections: How to Avoid Contagious Diseases.

ISBN 978-0-9982054-1-0, 978-0-9982054-0-3

Caribe ID, LLC and the Caribe ID Logo are trademarks of Caribe ID, LLC.

The information in this book is not intended as medical advice. The information provided is intended for your general knowledge and to stimulate conversation for you to ask questions of your healthcare providers. You should not use this information to diagnose or treat a health problem or disease without consulting with a qualified healthcare provider. Only your health care providers can diagnose and provide you with medical advice. Please consult with your physician regarding your individual situation prior to using any information gleaned from this book.

Table of Contents

≈

≈

ACKNOWLEDGEMENTS

For My Family and My Children

And Especially to Valarie

I Didn't Get This Far On My Own.

Brent W. Laartz, MD FIDSA

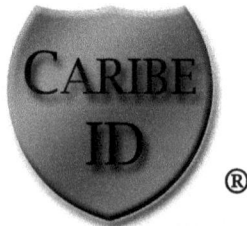

Publisher Caribe ID, LLC

Introduction

One early fall day, sailing on the waters of Tampa Bay, Florida with a friend, started me on this mission to educate people on how to avoid infections in healthcare settings and travel. You see, this friend had just returned a few months prior from a trip to Africa and he started to relate to me how he had developed a small rash on his foot that bothered him. Interspersed in this conversation, he complained about how healthcare was all about money and the feeling he had lost touch with his medical providers and insurance companies. It took hours for him to explain (and for me to question and understand) his other symptoms that were bothering him. He probably would not have told his healthcare providers about his anal itching and his chronic cough because he would not have thought them to be important. I helped him get tested for strongyloidiasis, which is a parasitic worm found throughout the world. Simple prevention techniques could have avoided this infection, but also basic knowledge of different diseases and conditions could have helped him navigate the healthcare system for a quicker diagnosis, in light of two providers having missed the diagnosis prior.

Since the beginning of the industrial revolution, man has been searching for ways to prevent infections. We have been through centuries of pestilence, from the Bubonic plague to cholera and influenza, and then to modern scourges, such as methicillin resistant staphylococcus aureus (MRSA), Escherichia coli (E coli), the continued prevalence of influenza, and now more recently with Ebola and Zika Virus outbreaks. In the era of modern medicine, physicians have been less eager to adopt infection illness prevention into their medical care. The general population has almost always been uninformed concerning even the simplest ways to protect themselves; this has largely been due to lack of communication from

1

healthcare providers. We seek advice mostly from mothers and friends perhaps because these are the most accessible sources.

As with any subject, misinformation is a common issue. People thought that putting flowers in their pockets would ward off the Black Plague, and tobacco was thought to prevent the illness. Children were made to smoke pipes at school in London because it was rumored that no tobacco shop owners had contracted the disease. During the influenza epidemic of 1918 millions of people died, but it was widely thought that bathing in an onion bath or wearing a goose grease poultice would ward off the disease. There were some semi-accurate teachings during this epidemic such as wearing masks, closing schools, and holding church services outside where there was more ventilation, but these activities were infrequently performed, unlike the different ineffective snake oils sold during those days.

In early to mid-nineteenth century London, the dawn of infection prevention started when John Snow discovered that, by removing the pump handle from the Broad Street water pump, he was able to limit a cholera outbreak that he determined was due to the location of the pump too close to untreated sewage. He was right in his beliefs that his actions could have a disease preventative impact, and he saved thousands of lives because of it. This fact that we have the power to protect ourselves from what previously was thought to be God's wrath, bad humors, or other supernatural powers, has been a relatively recent belief in our history.

Around the same time in Vienna, Austria, Dr. Ignaz Semmelweis held a theory that hand washing and using washed white lab coats during childbirth would prevent postpartum sepsis, an illness that claimed millions of new mothers prior to the age of modern medicine. He was ostracized by the medical community at the time, but eventually the use of hand washing techniques became the standard of care 30 years after his death. However, it continues to be a struggle for administrators of hospitals to improve handwashing compliance among nurses, doctors and other healthcare providers. At even the best hospitals, in surveillance studies, sometimes only 30% of doctors are washing their hands and 60% of nurses are washing their hands. Perhaps not so surprisingly, in one study, the most compliant healthcare workers were the housekeeping or dietary staff.

From the twentieth century to present day, the medical community has continued to communicate unproven and unscientific ways to prevent infections, while failing to communicate proven ways to prevent infection. As mentioned prior, in the past century there were widespread recommendations from doctors to patients about the use of goose grease poultices, onions, and garlic to prevent influenza. Even today, patients are not instructed to use proven methods to prevent post-surgical infections, such as simple topical treatments that can be used prior to surgery. Simple advice prior to travel is seldom given that could prevent travel related infections. At best it is glossed over in the hurry of a routine doctor's visit. Sometimes shockingly, nurses and doctors do not heed their own rational advice and continue to go to work when they are ill, possibly to the detriment of their patients.

There are 157,000 surgical site infections per year in the US, 722,000 hospital acquired infections with 75,000 deaths due to preventable infections secondary to exposure in the healthcare industry, whether it is hospitals, nursing facilities, rehabilitation facilities, or doctor's offices. There are many rather simple and seemingly obvious strategies that you can employ to protect yourself from what is often a deficient health care system when it comes to infection prevention. Some of these strategies involve being informed about your healthcare decisions and arming yourself with this information to become an advocate for your own safety. This book aims to inform you of these strategies to navigate the healthcare system and protect yourself from most scourges imaginable.

Our society has become more open, faraway lands are now more accessible, and our travels take us to the farthest reaches of the earth. But inherent in this freedom to trot the globe, we are also exposed to illnesses which we often don't think about and so often we do not consult a medical provider. Often our medical provider is not informed about methods to prevent these infections! Approximately 40% of all foreign travelers will experience a travel-related infection, and many of these are preventable. Some are not as serious, such as Montezuma's revenge (or traveler's diarrhea), that will only cause a 3 day interruption of your paradise vacation. However, there are potentially deadly infections that occur every day in US travelers to other exotic locations such as nearby Mexico and faraway Africa and Asia. Yellow Fever is in a group of viruses called Flaviviridae, and more recent similar viruses such as West Nile Virus, Dengue, and now Chikungunya and Zika virus are being diagnosed in travellers which could have potentially disabling long term effects.

This book's purpose is to inform the general public on ways to prevent various infections in their daily lives. Special emphasis is placed on prevention of MRSA infections, foodborne illnesses, viral infections, post-surgical infections, travel related infections such as malaria and dengue fever, and more communicable diseases such as Ebola and epidemic (such as Avian) influenza. While all of the scientific studies will be cited, I will attempt to limit the complete and sometimes boring medical lingo in favor of explanation of the subject in simpler terms that everyone can understand. In addition, this book favors vaccinations, in almost every chapter, from prevention of diseases during travel to prevention of pneumonia, influenza, STDs, and meningitis.

For more than a decade I have been the Director of Infection Control at one of the premier hospitals in the Tampa Bay area. Our infection rates are better than most of the area hospitals. Why, you ask? Because our administration and staff have been open to using proven infection control techniques with cost being a lesser concern. The small cost of a vigorous infection control program pays for itself, directly with decreased expenses and indirectly with improved patient outcomes. Some hospitals have been resistant to anything except surveillance and investigations of past outbreaks. Ninety-nine percent of all hospitals have a targeted screening program to assess whether patients have colonization with MRSA. This is because MRSA infections in hospitals are reduced by 20-40% by putting patients who have MRSA found in their noses in precautions. Precautions means that nurses, doctors, and visitors have to wear gowns and gloves while in the room. Hospitals which do not have these screening programs and more vigorous prevention programs are being "pound foolish" and may be risking the health of their patients. In addition, proactive hand-washing education on a regular basis, not just once a year, has been shown to be more effective.

Even with the best infection control programs, it is difficult for the hospital to prevent infections without your help. Likewise, your doctor is usually not aware of the required information nor has the time it takes to provide this knowledge to you. It is time for you to take control of your own destiny and learn how to protect yourself from basic infections from your home to the hospital and from the bedroom to beaches around the world. The methods you learned from your mother can sometimes direct you, however, to be better informed, you can start with this book. From within these pages you can start a dialogue with your healthcare providers so you can understand how preventive measures work, and more about the diseases and conditions themselves.

This book is not meant to be complete medical advice, which can only come from your healthcare provider. The information in this book is designed to educate you on each of these diseases and point you in the right direction so that you can discuss with your physician what will best work for you, the individual patient. Each person's infection risk is different, which is why this book is lengthy. There are parts of this book that will not apply to you, but you could use it to help a friend who has these individual health risks.

Ultimately, in the final chapter, I will list 25 things everyone can do to reduce their risk of infection every day. It can't get much simpler than that. Consider yourself protected, as much as you can do for yourself, that is.

John Snow and Cholera. **http://www.ph.ucla.edu/epi/snow/snowcricketarticle.html**

Hint: click on the yellow and green boxes on this website: **http://www.ph.ucla.edu/epi/snow.html**

Chapter 1

◠

Hospital Acquired Infections

Each year in the United States 589,000 people die of cancer, 377,000 die of heart disease and 356,000 die of other preventable health-care related events. Although some information is made public, now more than ever the press related to these events should be front-page news. These may be adverse events from medications, medical errors, or healthcare acquired infections. Approximately 722,000 people acquire a hospital related infection and 75,000 people die annually as a result. Not all healthcare infections are preventable, just as not all medication adverse events can be prevented. However, it is certainly true that not everything is being done to prevent these infections. It is estimated that, depending on the study, 20-70% of infections in hospitals are preventable.

I remember as though it were yesterday one of my first patients. She had just undergone a knee replacement several months earlier and now had an open wound with drainage that ultimately grew MRSA (Methicillin Resistant *Staphylococcus aureus*). Her orthopedic surgeon had told her that it was not an infection and that she did not need surgery. We gave her multiple rounds of intravenous antibiotics and tried to refer her to an orthopedic specialist in knee joint infections. She developed severe leg swelling (lymphedema) from the infections and had severe debility because of it. She became progressively weaker. I reflect on her often when I think about infection control, because it is these kinds of infections that we, as Hospital Epidemiologists, are trying to prevent.

Although the Center for Disease Control (CDC) uses the National Healthcare Safety Network (NHSN) to track these infections nationwide, it relies on hospitals to track their own rates of infection. This is seemingly like allowing the fox to guard the hen house. The rates are publicized; however, there are methods that hospitals can use to discount an infection and state that it was not really an infection. These methods are becoming less available as reporting loopholes are closed, but I have personally seen monthly rates at some hospitals that cannot be possible with the infections that I have personally seen during that previous month. To find out the infection rates at your local hospital, you can search the results at the NHSN website listed at the end of the chapter. There is also Medicare's database called Hospital Compare.

Among the different types of infections that can be acquired in hospitals are pneumonia, *Clostridium difficile* diarrhea, urinary tract infections, surgical site infections, and catheter related bloodstream infections. Some of the bacteria involved in these infections are already located on or in the body of the patient involved, but most are deposited onto the patient by healthcare workers or acquired from the environment of the hospital. The key to prevention lies with you monitoring these healthcare providers and being attuned to the cleanliness of your environment to assure your own safety. Please also see the 5 chapters on these individual entities for more information. Your immediate environment and the healthcare workers caring for you will protect your health but also pose the dangers of which you need to be aware.

The environment of a hospital room consists of a bed, the tray table, a bedside table, an IV pole, curtains, a bathroom and the floor. Prior to your arrival the staff perform a "terminal" clean which is the most thorough clean this room will have during your stay. This thorough clean is highly variable and at most hospitals is less than adequate. The maintenance staff is supposed to clean all surfaces and allow the cleaner to remain wet on all surfaces for 3-10 minutes (depending on the product), which is the kill time for many bacteria. However, in studies, testing these surfaces shows that less than 50% of the surfaces are truly cleaned and up to 90% of surveillance cultures after this clean had growth of enteric (intestinal type) bacteria. This includes operating rooms, hospital rooms, and pharmacy clean rooms.

Hospitals have access to monitoring equipment to educate and monitor the cleanliness of this terminal clean. If done right, a simple ATP testing machine can provide immediate feedback and is cheaper than surveillance equipment, which would require culturing swabs from hundreds of samples. It is from this information that it becomes painfully obvious that hospitals are not clean unless routine assessment and education are done for the housekeeping staff. The best hospitals use this type of immediate feedback machine to validate the housekeeper's cleaning job. However, very few hospitals use this equipment. Therefore it is up to you to protect yourself by making the assessments and, if necessary, cleaning your environment for your own safety.

Each day, high contact surfaces should be cleaned thoroughly with a solution that kills bacteria and viruses effectively. This includes the tray tables, bed rails, bedside table, IV poles and bathroom. If you think the terminal clean is poor, just imagine what the daily clean percent coverage is. Similar to the terminal clean the surfaces should be wet for 10 minutes to assure killing of the bacteria that could, if left unchecked, reach your wound or your IV catheter or become ingested after you touch it.

It will be up to you to verify the cleanliness of your room and to supervise all of the cleanings. It may come as a shock, but after you monitor the cleaning for a short time, you will come to realize that you may need to do some cleaning yourself! When you first arrive in the Emergency Room, exam room, or your inpatient room, inspect the room. At first glance, it will appear clean. However, look a little closer. Watch the staff as they clean to assess the adequacy of their cleaning. If you are concerned about the cleanliness of your room, then buy your own canister of bleach cleaning wipes. These bleach cleaning wipes are hard on the surfaces of hospitals and this is why they are not used routinely by hospital staff. However, you as a patient should not have to worry about this. It is wise to have family with you when you arrive and for most of the day each day you are in the hospital since you may be too weak to do the necessary cleaning. All touch surfaces on the bed rail, tray table, bedside table, and IV pole should be cleaned. If you are going to sit in the chair, it should be cleaned. The call light/television control should be cleaned and any other objects that the patient will handle and are not disposable should be cleaned. The IV pole and IV pump should be cleaned. Now, on a daily basis or more often, repeat this clean with the bleach wipes. Be aware that you should use gloves and be careful about the fumes from bleach products, since some people are sensitive to them. Never use bleach wipes in combination with another cleaner.

Any toiletry area should also be thoroughly cleaned including the sink and faucet handles. Healthcare personnel should not be using the sink to dump urine or dirty materials like wash basins because they will need to wash their hands there and the sink will be the source of water for your daily bath. All of these materials need to be disposed of in the toilet or in a soiled utility room nearby. Make sure the sink is as clean as possible. There are multiple studies showing hospital infection outbreaks related to sinks. You should monitor the cleaning and request cleaning more often if you see anyone dumping dirty materials in the sink. At one of our hospitals we thoroughly clean the sink daily. To prevent growth of bacteria in the drain and trap we dump 250 ml of vinegar in the drain daily and let it sit.

In other chapters I will mention hand washing compliance. It is completely on purpose that I duplicate this information so much in this book. This subject is SO important that it needs to be touched on again and again and AGAIN!! Study after study has shown that hospitals that have recently had consistent hand hygiene interventions see their infection rates plummet. However, the rates of both hand washing and infections may not stay respectable for long, as the education push becomes quickly forgotten. At one hospital I like to have monthly infection control rounds on each of the floors and hand hygiene compliance is always better when we do this. This intervention kept the concept of 100% compliance with hand sanitization on the nurse's minds consistently. The best interventions are those that have daily or weekly reminders that constantly prompt nurses and physicians and other staff to wash their hands.

Even better interventions are daily reminders by you, the patient! When you get to your room, ask for an extra canister or bottle of the alcohol-based hand sanitizer that usually is in a container hung on a wall by the door. Place this bottle on the tray table of your room. The only caveat to this is if your family member has dementia or delirium and may try to ingest the sanitizer. Then, obviously this will not be a good idea. If you do not see a healthcare provider cleanse their hands, it is possible that they did it from a canister outside the door, but it is not considered rude for you to hold the canister out toward the individual without saying anything. This is a good way to provide a non-shaming reminder. You should also use it frequently on your own hands and the hands of any guests you may have.

Other facility healthcare workers should feel empowered to teach others when they observe others not sanitizing their hands. Watch for this type of attitude rather than the "look the other way" attitude that has been pervasive in our healthcare systems. A hospital with a teamwork attitude that protects you, the patient, is far better than hospitals with a lack of quality control. Watch for continuous teaching among all of the providers and healthcare personnel.

Watch for the consistent use of gloves when handling IV's and wounds. There should be no reason to touch an area of potential infection, such as the end of an IV, a wound, or a Foley urinary catheter without wearing gloves. When changing fluids or intravenous medication bags, both the IV connector going into the patient and the new tubing connector need to be wiped with either an alcohol prep pad or other cleaning method.

Bathing of patients, peri-care (cleaning of the groin and buttocks area), incontinence management, and decubitus ulcer or bedsore prevention are some of the most important jobs in the arena of nursing and nursing technician responsibilities. Bathing can be a very important way of decreasing the amount of bacteria on the skin of patients. In one instance, we were astonished to discover that the "tech" was washing the groin first then moving to the rest of the body and face with the same washcloth and washbasin. Family members would be able to spot this easily if they are looking for it. Management of incontinence and bathing quickly after bowel movements can prevent urine infections, decubitus ulcers, and surgical wound infections. To protect yourself here, you will need to have a family member monitor bathing closely. Some family members take a proactive stance with helping clean their own loved ones. It is these patients who rarely have a decubitus ulcer, even with the most immobile of patients.

Indwelling urinary catheters represent the easiest pathway for bacteria to enter the body during your hospital stay. The occurrence of an infection while you have a catheter (which was not present on admission) is a actionable event. Thus hospitals have protocols in place to prevent them. At all times there should be an assessment as to the continued need for the urinary catheter. If you are able to get to a commode, there should be no need for one unless there is an urine flow obstruction or something called urinary retention. On the other hand, for incontinent, immobile patients, a catheter could help prevent decubitus ulcers because it prevents pooling of urine in the bed near the buttocks. A decision between the need for the catheter and removing it must be made. In addition, during the insertion of the catheter, all care to make the area as clean as possible must be exercised.

When looking at the compliance of hospital staff to perform standard of care precautions during insertion and maintenance of a urinary catheter, it is usually around 30% for all infection prevention measures. The Foley catheter needs to be placed in a hygienic fashion, cleaning the area with a special soap, and inserting without touching any other surfaces. The bag needs to be lower than the body and there should be no "dependent loop," which is a U shaped dip in the tube that goes below the level of the urine in the bag. The U shape is smaller if the catheter is placed farther from the groin, such as near the feet. There are a multitude of other risk factors for urinary tract infections that can be mitigated, and these are mentioned in the document listed at the end of the chapter and in the chapter on urinary tract infections.

I cringe whenever I walk into a room and I see a patient lying with the head of the bed down flat or worse yet, the head of the bed is at the required 30 degrees, but their head is wedged between the bed and the bedrail where the flat part of the bed meets the angled part. This is a recipe for disaster, and that disaster is pneumonia. The recipe for pneumonia involves the ingredients of aspiration and immobility. When a person is bedridden in the hospital, the lungs are not expanded adequately because, when lying down, the person cannot breathe deeply enough to open the smallest airways. When this occurs, pooling of secretions occurs in the base of the lungs and it is more difficult for the body to clear these secretions. In addition, when a person is very weak it is difficult to prevent saliva and food from going from the mouth to the lungs. This is called aspiration.

In order to prevent pneumonia, hospitals utilize prevention protocols. The more you can understand these prevention techniques, the better. Incentive spirometers are devices that, when used along with deep breathing exercises, directed cough, early ambulation, and optimal pain relief, have been shown to decrease pulmonary complications of certain hospitalized patients. Incentive spirometers should be used 10 times every hour. Inhaling against the pressure of the device causes the small airways to expand. Some immobile patients should have a respiratory technician supervise a directed cough, forcefully coughing in a "huff cough" periodically, and active deep breathing exercises. To prevent aspiration, the head of the bed should be raised to at least 30-45 degrees, and aspiration precautions should be used for all weakened patients. Aspiration precautions involve sitting straight up (90 degrees) when eating or drinking, avoiding the use of a straw, and tilting the chin down towards the chest for every swallow.

Another way to prevent pneumonia is to become as mobile as you can when it is safe to do so. When confined to bed, exercise arm and leg muscles if your nurse or physician says you are allowed. If you sit up in bed your lungs will expand more and you should ask if you could sit in a chair as much as possible. All too many people expect that they should just stay in bed (sometimes rightfully so if pain or wounds prevent mobility) and these immobile patients are more likely to develop complications. However, if you have a surgical wound, be aware to not stretch the edges too much. This especially applies when you have an abdominal wound, getting up will place pressure on the sides of the wound. If you are sitting up or standing up, be sure not to use your abdominal muscles to do so. Early ambulation is important if it is under supervision of your doctor, nurse, and physical therapist.

Nutrition is also important for prevention of wound infections and pneumonia. If you regain appetite and the ability to take in nutrition more quickly, you will be able to regain mobility sooner. Listen to your physicians and nurses and request a dietitian as soon as possible during your hospital stay. For the sickest patients, intravenous nutrition or nutrition through a feeding tube into the stomach or small bowel may be appropriate. Early use of these forms of nutrition has been shown to improve outcomes in the intensive care unit.

An important concept that is becoming more apparent is monitoring for "Failure to Resuscitate". There is a lot of data that says that it is not necessarily the complication rate that leads to the worst outcomes. The complication rate may have a lot to do with the complexity of the cases involved, therefore complication rates are not the best metric by which to measure hospitals. Recognition of complications early and making attempts at correcting those complications is called resuscitation. It is this recognition that will save your life since complications can and do happen. Watch your doctor to see if they take input from nurses well. If your nurse calls the doctor with a low or high blood pressure or fever, monitor the response. If it is not adequate, this could lead to problems. Watch to see if the doctor expects high quality reporting from all of the healthcare team. If they have a lackadaisical response this will not lead to as high quality outcomes as those with an aggressive monitoring of your progress.

The problem with today's healthcare safety monitoring programs is that they only measure complication rates such as infections. One past metric was to evaluate the occurrence of pneumonia in patients on ventilators, called ventilator-associated pneumonia (VAP). The metric was refined by the CDC since they recognized that the rate of infections almost completely disappeared once there was reporting to state and federal government programs. One could argue that the rates went down because of prevention efforts also, but the CDC was forced to redefine occurrences more strictly to catch infections. Surgical skin infections could be called seromas and hematomas, instead of the potential infections that they are, and thus escape reporting. Every year hospitals are required to send to surgeons a survey to report all post-surgical infections. Every year those surveys come back with zero rates of infections. This doesn't seem plausible. Another method to avoid reporting of infection complications could be to admit the infected patient to a different hospital than the one in which the procedure was performed. Most hospitals will avoid reporting all but the most obvious cases to the other hospital, though at reputable hospitals this tactic is disappearing.

So one can easily see how the system provides negative incentives to a physician for accurately reporting an infection. However, this could lead to disastrous consequences if the infection is ignored and not treated adequately. There are no positive incentives for recognizing an infection early and treating it appropriately, only the negative consequence of the infection. Be your own advocate when it comes to reporting fevers, redness or drainage around your wound, or any other sign of infection. Report this not only to your surgeon but also report it to your primary care physician and anyone else you can find. There are wound care center physicians who often treat infections in surgical wounds and they are often an advocate for your quality treatment.

It is important to become your family member's or your own advocate and monitor in the hospital. If you will not be in the room for any period of time, it will be important for your loved one to be able to get in touch with you from their hospital room. Place your phone number on the whiteboard and on the tray table in front of them with large numbers that are easy to read. Provide a cell phone if necessary since hospital telephones are very confusing for someone who may already be confused from being ill.

Additional Information:

National Health Safety Network: **http://www.cdc.gov/nhsn/**

Hospital Compare: **https://www.cms.gov/medicare/quality-initiatives-patient-assessment-instruments/hospitalqualityinits/hospitalcompare.html**

https://www.apic.org/Resource /EliminationGuideForm/0ff6ae59-0a3a-4640-97b5-eee38b8bed5b/File/CAUTI 06.pdf

Chapter 2

∼

Rehabilitation Centers and Skilled Nursing Facilities

Despite the attention placed on the issue by doctors, nurses, and administrators, infections in rehabilitation centers and skilled nursing facilities (SNF) remain one of the most important problems in infection control today. These facilities are notoriously underfunded by their reimbursements and therefore have very little excess money to implement infection control programs. Their infection control programs are often run by an experienced, but not necessarily infection control trained, nurse in the facility. To add to the problem, the facility residents are often weakened by the illnesses that required their admission and are at risk for a multitude of infections including aspiration pneumonia, decubitus ulcers (bed sores), and urinary tract infections. Unlike hospitals, there are often inadequate programs to limit Foley catheters or to decrease the risk of aspiration pneumonia, though this is changing. Due to facility credentialing and legal ramifications, they usually have good prevention strategies for decubitus ulcers but the methods are not universal and many are too understaffed to implement them fully.

I have personally seen many cases of obvious nursing home neglect, usually in the form of multiple decubitus ulcer wounds. However, the real silent epidemic is the infections occurring as a result of less than adequate infection control. For example, remember vividly the frail elderly lady with Norovirus diarrhea after an outbreak in the nursing facility that was still not recognized at the time of her admission. I have also seen countless surgical wound infections acquired after being discharged to the nursing facility. For a short period of time many years ago, I was an infection control director for a nursing facility. As a result I have tried to assess the adequacy of infection control in these centers through interviewing patients in the hospital and have come to some concrete conclusions. Because the challenge of infection control in the nursing facility may be too complex for them to manage, it is crucial for the patient or the patient's family to take an active role in prevention.

Let us separate this chapter by the different illnesses that commonly occur in rehab facilities and discuss each separately. The issue of assigning blame is often a confusing one because the residents are weakened and contribute a high proportion of risk. The same issues of hand washing and cleanliness from hospitals occur in rehab facilities but with even less compliance. Extreme skin care vigilance for ulcer prevention, wound care, as well as programs to increase mobility and turning of patients in bed who are unable to move are all extremely important.

One issue with controlling SNF infections stems from patients' movement throughout the facility areas. In hospitals patients are, for the most part, confined to their rooms. In rehab facilities there are common dining rooms, bathrooms, gyms, smoking areas and patios. Cleaning these areas after use is usually spotty at best. The patients are often not isolated for communicable diseases as stringently as in hospitals. Consequently, one person who was just discharged from the hospital for MRSA pneumonia could use a piece of equipment in the gym, followed by a patient who had just undergone a total hip arthroplasty and therefore has a vulnerable wound. This will be the single most important situation to avoid.

Cleanliness and hand washing are the keys to avoiding MRSA infections in the rehab facility. Be hypervigilant about the adequacy of cleaning and if you notice the environment is not adequately cleaned, raise your concerns to the supervisors to change their practices. If this does not work, then bring your own antibacterial wipes and use them in your room on what is called high touch areas. This includes any tables, IV poles, trays, bed rails, and sinks. An additional area of risk is the gym. Bring the same wipes there and use them on the equipment if you notice they do not adequately clean in between patients. Have family members assist with this, if necessary. Monitor the effectiveness of the staff's hand sanitation.

Alcohol foam dispensers are best, but soap and water should also be used. Ask for an extra foam or alcohol gel dispenser and place it on your tray table. Use it for your own hands several times daily and you can offer it to staff that you notice have not washed theirs. The exception to leaving this alcohol gel on the table obviously is if your loved one has dementia and could potentially ingest the foam or gel.

Skin infections from MRSA and other bacteria are common in rehab facilities for more than one reason. Some risk factors present in elderly patients include thin skin, poor nutrition, edema or swelling, weakness, diabetes and peripheral vascular disease. Older patients are often weak, needing to be transferred from their bed to the wheelchair or assisted out of bed by belts and lifts. These lifts can shear against the thinner skin of an elderly patient causing skin tears and wounds. Nutritional deficiencies are common in rehab patients that can cause thin skin and edema. Diabetes and peripheral vascular disease cause an increased risk for wounds and infection. Poor healing can result from immune suppressant medications that are commonly given to the elderly, especially corticosteroids like prednisone.

Arising from these issues are the decubitus ulcers. These are also called pressure ulcers or bed sores. The pressure of lying on a bony prominence such as the sacrum, the hip or the heel causes decreased blood flow and tissue damage. This causes a blister to form and once this opens the wound can get infected. Urinary incontinence is a large risk factor for decubitus ulcers of the sacrum, ischium and hip area. Keeping the skin dry helps prevent opportunities for skin breakdown and possible infection. If there is lack of mobility there should be frequent turning the patient in bed. This involves turning from side to side often at least every two hours.

Protective devices for the feet, elbows and knees are available to take pressure off an area. These are called heel or elbow protectors and you may need to ask for them if the heels or elbows are immobilized and sit with pressure on the bed. A pillow under the calves is slightly less effective but can be used if there are no heel protectors available. If lying on the side, a pillow between the knees and ankles should be used because the pressure of one ankle or leg lying on top of the other creates wounds. Specialized beds should be requested if there is a significant amount of time spent in bed. Sometimes decubitus ulcers are difficult to avoid if there is extreme lack of mobility as in severe dementia and contracted patients.

Urinary tract infections (UTI's) are frequent in nursing and rehab facilities partially due to the use of Foley catheters, but also owing to the weakness of an individual's skeletal and bladder muscles. This weakness may cause incomplete bladder emptying and the resulting in increased risk of UTI. If a patient cannot get up to go to the bathroom and patient care techs are not available to bring a bedpan or assist the patient in getting up to the commode, incontinence or UTI may result. In addition, cleaning of the groin area may be less than adequate due to understaffing. Dehydration due to poor intake or inadequate provision of liquids could lead to increased risk. Most quality institutions have implemented policies for adequate hydration, bowel care and cleaning, and incontinence rounds. Please see the chapter on protection from UTI's for more specific information.

Pneumonia, influenza and other respiratory infections such as metapneumovirus and respiratory syncytial virus (RSV) are common, and outbreaks may occur in nursing facilities many times during the year. Viral outbreaks are difficult to control in nursing facilities due to the same issues outlined prior. If one person contracts a viral infection it may not be possible to prevent further infections with the close quarters of a nursing facility. However, it should be possible to limit the number of infections as soon as it is determined there is a viral respiratory infection issue. This is important because 10-20% of viral infections in the elderly result in pneumonia, one of the top killers of senior citizens.

Viruses spread through both contact and respiratory droplets, which means they spread within three to six feet of the sick individual. Some viruses are airborne and can spread up to 20 feet. Because of this, when there is an initial occurrence of any respiratory viral illness in a nursing facility, a complete cleaning program needs to be undertaken, including the nursing staff areas. This activity needs to be frequently performed until three days have gone by without a new illness. However, recognition of the viral infections is important. I have seen hospitals, nursing facilities and rehab facilities that wait until three or more cases are identified before they acknowledge an outbreak. If the facility is in a hospital it is usually detected more quickly because the diagnosis is made sooner. Also, any staff that becomes ill with fever, upper respiratory symptoms such as cough, or diarrhea needs to not come to work, period. If there is influenza in the facility, it is reasonable to institute a preventive influenza medication called oseltamivir at least until the outbreak is over or the end of the influenza season, and consider giving at-risk individuals influenza vaccinations if they have not received it for the year. Outside of a nursing facility the duration of preventive treatment is 10 days. The duration of preventive treatment is longer in a nursing facility and usually is from the start of the first case until 10 days after the last case is diagnosed. It usually takes about two weeks for flu vaccine to provide protection for persons; it may not prevent the occurrence of the flu, but will make the flu milder and prevent death.

Diarrheal illnesses are also common in these facilities such as rotavirus, norovirus (from cruise ship fame), *E. coli*, *Salmonella* and *Clostridium difficile*. Rotavirus and Norovirus are viruses that can be spread easily from one person to another by contact with either the sick individual or anything the sick individual has touched. These outbreaks are even harder to stop than viral respiratory illnesses because the attack rate (the percentage of exposed individuals who become ill) is higher. This is why large numbers of passengers on a cruise ship can become ill. Every winter and spring there are norovirus outbreaks in nursing facilities, hospitals and outpatient facilities. Every year many go unnoticed and unchecked. The good thing is less people die from a viral gastroenteritis outbreak than a viral respiratory outbreak. However, the weakness that comes from the illness could predispose the elderly to other infections that are fatal such as pneumonia. Again, be aware of the symptoms of the patients around you. Equally important is the health of the staff because many Norovirus outbreaks are started or continued by staff that become ill with the virus. During these outbreaks there should be hourly deep cleaning with appropriate cleaning products around the clock.

Clostridium difficile (C diff) is a bacterium that, due to frequent antibiotic usage in nursing facilities, is increasing in numbers. Unlike viral gastroenteritis, the mortality rate is up to 10% or more in the elderly. One in 11 people older than 65 died within a month of C diff diagnosis and more than 80% of C diff deaths occurred in people age 65 and older. The difficult situation is that spores (like seeds in plants) from C diff can remain on surfaces in the facility for months and remain on and in the body of the sick individual even after he is treated and asymptomatic. The spores can then be ingested just by touching a contaminated surface and eating with the same hands. These spores can only be eliminated by bleach cleaning of all contact surfaces or possibly by complete UV radiation. See the chapter on *Clostridium difficile* for more information.

The first step to protecting yourself from C diff infection begins with observation. Every effort should be given to visit loved ones in the nursing facility daily or weekly. Observe the cleanliness and bring your own bleach wipes and hand sanitizer if necessary. Leave a pump alcohol hand sanitizer on the bedside table as long as there is not severe dementia to the point they could ingest it. If the patient has mobility issues, some family members should participate in an extra bedside bathing if you see evidence that there is inattention to this. Feel empowered to request extra bathing. This is part of your right as a patient or family member. If there is an issue of mobility, be vigilant about decubitus prevention. If even the slightest bit of redness shows up on a pressure point, this is a stage I decubitus ulcer and you should request a wound care practitioner consult. The early intervention could prevent future infections.

To prevent urinary tract infections, make sure you or your loved one are always hydrated. Foley catheters should be used only sparingly and every attempt to not use them is important. With that said, if an immobile patient is incontinent the resulting wetness of the skin on the backside could promote development of decubitus ulcers, so be careful. Consult your physician. See the chapter on urinary tract infections for more ideas.

Monitor every other resident, especially a roommate, for any signs of a respiratory or diarrheal illness and make sure there is adequate cleaning. If you hear of a case of influenza, especially in a roommate, request a course of prophylactic (preventive) oseltamivir from your physician. It is reasonable to request a simple ear loop mask for your loved one to wear while in dining or gym areas. Bring your own mask if need be. If there is a diarrheal illness in the facility, bring your own cleaning materials such as bleach wipes to wipe down all surfaces daily (or more often) including the bathroom, tray table, bed rails and any other furniture your loved one might touch. Be careful if your loved ones have breathing difficulties as the fumes from bleach could precipitate some breathing difficulties. Also, wear gloves when using these wipes. The bacteria and viruses are there and the staff may not have the time to ensure your safety. Although this should all be done by the facility, if you want to protect yourself YOU must be the vigilant one. Additionally, make sure adequate immunization for *Streptococcus pneumoniae* and influenza have been given. See the chapter on influenza and pneumonia.

If your loved one has had *Clostridium difficile* in the past and is now better, be sure that they are taking probiotics if approved by your physician. Use gloves when you are cleaning because you could also ingest the spores and you don't want to use bleach wipes without gloves. If there are others in the facility who have had C diff (and there are, trust me), use the same precautions. Request to use bleach wipes before you or your family member uses the gym equipment.

If your loved one has a wound, request to be there when they are changing the dressing. Make sure the staff uses gloves. Request a wound care consult, as every nursing facility should have contracts with outside wound care agencies that have physician oversight.   Sometimes there is a dedicated wound care nurse in the facility. The wound care nurses that will come with this consult will have far better training than the general nursing staff at the facility.   If there is a hint of drainage, see your physician as soon as possible. Do not let a wound be soiled with urine or feces for long and request an immediate cleaning. Finally, be aware again of the dangers of the surrounding areas of the patient's environment and make sure they are clean. Remember, you are empowered to protect yourself.

Finally, be prepared to be a voice for your own safety. Speak up clearly with supervisors. Remember that only the squeaky wheel gets the grease, but be kind to the nurses as they are your best friends. They often are well intentioned but trapped in an inadequate system, working long hours. Pick a facility that has your own physician on staff or a physician well known to your primary care physician as they can also be an advocate for you.

Chapter 3

~

Methicillin Resistant Staphylococcus Aureus (MRSA) and Skin and Wound Infections

Those who have had MRSA infections will tell you about the change it brings, especially that having this bacterium changes them into a compulsive neat freak and none of this seems to work to prevent infection from occurring. While there are certain risk factors for developing MRSA skin infections, such as skin disorders or trauma, some infections occur in a completely normal, clean area of skin. Young, healthy people and children I have seen have had multiple recurrences with the same skin infection in different areas of their body. One young person I met started using a severe, unorthodox method of bathing using bleach causing harm to himself. He did this in the extreme attempt to rid his skin of this bacterium. There are, however, much safer ways to eradicate this scourge from your body.

MRSA has only been around for 40 years, but its origins come from the advent and subsequent overuse of antibiotics. With each wave of new antibiotics, starting with penicillin in the 1950's then aminopenicillins, methicillin, vancomycin, daptomycin, and linezolid, we have been over-confident about the battle against bacteria, especially *Staph aureus*, which causes skin infections, pneumonia, bone infections, and heart valve infections. In fact, in 1928, Sir Alexander Fleming, who discovered penicillin, said, "It seems likely that in the next few years a combination of antibiotics with different antibacterial spectra will furnish a "cribrum therapeuticum" (or therapeutic sieve) from which fewer and fewer bacteria will escape." This statement could not have been further from the truth. We now harbor no illusions that bacteria are completely defeatable. We have, however, done a masterful job at coming up with new ways of winning some infection battles. The discovery of new antibiotics is becoming less frequent resulting in a push to find the newest big guns for the infection war.

Methicillin-resistant *Staph aureus* has been one of the most challenging bacteria as the diseases it can cause are relatively difficult to treat. It causes simple skin abscesses that progress rapidly despite starting appropriate oral antibiotics. It invades rapidly and causes surgical site infections that can be rapidly fatal if not treated appropriately. It often requires intravenous antibiotics to eradicate. MRSA can also cause serious lung, heart valve, joint, and bone infections, some of which can become chronic infections requiring lifelong antibiotics. Such infections often require surgical excision of abscesses and the implanted devices.

What makes this bacterium difficult to treat is that it has mechanisms to stick to foreign materials, thus allowing it to adhere to hemodialysis catheters, central venous catheters in hospitals and surgical implants such as joint replacements and pacemakers. The difficulty in eradicating MRSA off these devices often requires lengthy hospital stays and multiple surgeries to remove the devices. As one can imagine it is no small feat to remove the artificial hip joint of an 80 year old to eradicate this bacterium. What if one bacterium remains in the area of the hip after you remove it? What if it survives the 6 weeks of intravenous antibiotics? For this reason, if it has been greater than 30 days after the surgery, removal can requires two or more surgeries.

Scientists have known about *Staphylococcus aureus* for decades as a bacterium commonly found on the skin. It can cause abscesses or boils and other skin infections. It was described by Ogsden in 1881. By the 1940s we had discovered penicillin, which eradicated staph infections, giving us a new big gun for these infections during World War II, but the bacteria became resistant by the end of the war. In the 1950s we discovered a new antibiotic called methicillin that killed *Staph aureus* better than any antibiotic. Within a few years we discovered that some staph could become resistant to it, hence the name methicillin-resistant *Staph aureus*. There are multipole strains of MRSA now: some hospital acquired (HA) and others community acquired (CA). Sometimes this naming system is arbitrary as one could acquire the CA strain anywhere, including in the hospital. The community acquired strains (with names like USA 100) are much more aggressive and cause large boils in healthy adults and children.

Any explanation on how to protect yourself from MRSA needs to include a discussion on colonization. As explained in a few other chapters, we are a cesspool of bacteria, . We have trillions of bacteria (and yeast) all over our bodies, outside and in some internal areas. This is absolutely normal. There are bacteria on the skin, especially staph and strep bacteria, but also intestinal bacteria in the areas around the groin and buttocks area. There are bacteria anywhere exposed to the intestines or the outside world: the bladder, vagina, penis, nose, sinuses, eyes, mouth, esophagus, stomach and intestines. The bacteria that exist on and in our bodies are called colonizing bacteria. Studies suggest that up to 40% of Americans are colonized with MRSA at any given time. MRSA is very opportunistic in that any opening in the skin, such as an ingrown hair, a small nick in the skin, or an open wound can allow the bacteria entry to cause a skin infection or worse. Given that we all sustain small, unnoticeable nicks in the skin on a daily basis, this is a potential ticking time bomb waiting to explode. If MRSA happens to be at the site of the tiny wound, it can invade. Once it invades it communicates with its offspring to start growing exponentially (called "quorum sensing"). A dime sized wound can become a softball sized abscess overnight. If this abscess is not surgically drained, it can kill in the matter a days.

We first started noticing these very aggressive strains of CA MRSA in the 1990s as large numbers of young adults and children began to present to their doctor with infections that seemed to defy the oral antibiotics that were prescribed for them. Children, especially, were spreading it among schools and daycares; however, it was uncommon in children of stay-at-home parents. Children's sometimes poor hygiene lent itself well for the spread of a skin-dwelling bacteria and soon the bacteria was widespread, causing numerous hospitalizations and costing the US healthcare system billions of dollars. There are more than 100,000 admissions per year in the US for skin infections, about half of which are due to MRSA.

Sports teams and locker rooms have become high profile locations to acquire MRSA colonization and infection due to the close proximity of players and injuries they sustain, accompanied by the lack of cleaning in the locker room. A simple case of turf toe or a bruise can result in an infection if MRSA is able to invade in the same area. Several professional sports teams in the US have been in the news for having multiple team members diagnosed with everything from simple skin infections to serious conditions like heart valve and bone infections contracted through locker room contamination. I've seen some very highly paid athletes never regain complete use of a shoulder or knee due to a MRSA infection after what was supposed to be a career resurrecting surgery.

The danger of MRSA lies in its ability to invade deeper. If the skin infection or boil is close to a bone or joint, it can cause a bone infection called osteomyelitis or a joint infection called septic arthritis. If MRSA invades into the bloodstream it can travel to a remote site and cause a heart valve infection (endocarditis) or a bone or joint infection, most commonly in the spine (vertebral osteomyelitis). All of these deeper infections require prolonged courses (6 to 8 weeks) of intravenous antibiotics to eradicate. They also commonly require surgery to drain the pus pockets or remove parts of infected bone.

This invasion can occur from an innocent looking wound that becomes infected by bacteria such as MRSA that is on the surrounding skin. I was asked just the other day by a sweet, elderly lady who had an infected cat scratch, "How did I get this bacteria? I am very clean and have a clean house." Clearly from the patients I have seen, it is often not their cleanliness (though sometimes it is) but just bad luck to have a small break in the skin in the wrong spot where the MRSA is lurking.

Thus the key to prevention of MRSA skin infections is to monitor any open areas of skin and clean them appropriately. Some people are more prone to have a disrupted skin barrier, such as those with psoriasis, atopic dermatitis, or chronic athlete's foot. Edema (extra fluid that collects in the tissues) could also cause open areas that would allow bacteria under the skin. Because of these and other possible factors, some people experience multiple episodes of MRSA skin infections. I have seen patients with monthly infections and, as mentioned before, these patients become the most obsessive clean freaks yet nothing they do prior to visiting me has helped prevent the infections. Though many think so, rarely is this infection due to the bacteria being harbored inside the body. It could be that they remain colonized with MRSA and then get a new infection in a new location or they become re-colonized with MRSA from a source such as a family member, a family pet, or something in their home or community. Given the fact that 40% of people are colonized with MRSA they could re-acquire it anywhere.

For those who have multiple infections with MRSA I usually recommend decolonization. I do not recommend it for everyone with MRSA infections because overuse of the decolonization regimen could induce resistance to the agents. The regimen consists of daily head to toe baths with 2% chlorhexidine soap and topical mupirocin ointment to each nostril twice daily for 5 days. Depending on the circumstances, I may have them do a longer course for 30 days after which I have them perform the regimen for the first week of every month for a few months or longer. Mupirocin is only obtainable by prescription. They also need to follow a regimen of bathroom, kitchen, linens and clothes cleaning during the period of decolonization. Personal care areas (but not your body!!) should be cleaned with a diluted (10%) bleach solution. Clothes and linens should be cleaned in hot water. It may fade some clothes but helps decrease the amount of bacteria on the clothes and linens. Sometimes I recommend family or pets have the same treatments, especially if any of them have had skin infections.

If you have had a boil or other infection with MRSA, avoid reusing or sharing personal care items such as razors, brushes, makeup brushes, lipstick, etc. Anything that you use on your skin should be disposed of and replaced. Areas of the skin that become wet frequently should be dried often. Take measures to prevent ongoing wetness such as wearing dry wicking socks or bras. If you have psoriasis or eczema, try to optimize the treatment by seeing a dermatologist. Use alcohol gel to sanitize your hands frequently. While not proven, I might try to avoid shaving completely down to the skin and only use clippers to bring down to a short hair height. The rationale for my thinking is that shaving in an area before a surgical procedure used to be done regularly until it was found to increase infections.

MRSA is not the only bacterium that causes cellulitis or skin infections. *Streptococcus* and *Pseudomonas* species are the next most common after staphylococcus. These bacteria love warm, moist places so they often start at the feet where there is often moistness between the toes. *Pseudomonas* can be found in tennis shoes and hot tubs, for example. In general the same principles hold here as for MRSA, except there are no decolonization regimens. Any open cut and any significant fungal infections of the feet should be cared for immediately.

Some persons with lymphedema (chronic edema) are at risk for recurrent rapid *Strep* skin infections. This is because *Streptococcus* bacteria, which commonly enter the skin at tiny nicks and cuts, are eradicated on a daily basis by the same lymphatic system that is blocked in lymphedema. Lymphedema is caused by damage to the lymph vessels or lymph nodes possibly due to surgery in the pelvis, breast or axilla that often accompanies cancer treatments such as radiation, or pelvic trauma. Lymphedema treatments such as sleeves or lymphedema pumps may help some but these are useful mainly to ameliorate the symptoms of swelling associated with the condition. Because it is almost always associated with *Strep* bacteria, taking cephalexin or penicillin can prevent infection if you have had recurrent infections associated with lymphedema. Taken once or twice daily, the antibiotic prevents the strep bacteria from invading and the bacteria never becomes resistant. I usually only give this preventive treatment to patients who have more than one or two infections per year.

There is a condition called hidradenitis suppurativa that is common in those with frequent skin infections, especially in the underarm, groin and breast areas. The condition is caused by abnormal sweat glands. It is seen more often in obese patients and those with diabetes. These people often describe foul smelling wounds in these areas which have a scarred appearance. Weight loss usually decreases the severity and frequency of infections. Seeing a wound care specialist or dermatologist is key to the control.

Two special bacteria from water exposure are *Vibrio vulnificus* and *Aeromonas* from salt and fresh water respectively. Also cat and dog exposures can lead to *Pasteurella* or *Capnocytophaga* infections. Soil or plant exposure could lead to *Nocardia* infections that look like nodules travelling up the limb. Slow growing infections after surgery or with exposure to soil or salt water could be caused by *Mycobacteria* which are detected by special cultures that are not performed routinely. If you have a skin infection after a certain exposure, make sure you tell your physician about the possible exposures no matter how trivial you think the exposure may have been. All of the bacteria caused by these exposures require special antibiotics not usually used for skin infections.

Now let's learn more about how to protect yourself from these infections in wounds. The key to wound care relates to getting the healing factors and oxygen from the bloodstream to the wound and keeping bacterial colonization to a minimum. For prevention of surgical wound infections, please see the chapter on surgical wound infections. Many of the same principles apply to all wounds regarding diabetes, obesity, peripheral vascular disease, and smoking. Elevated blood sugar levels (even mildly elevated) cause poisoning of the infection-fighting white blood cells and the healing repair cells in the skin. It also causes blood supply issues by narrowing the small blood vessels in the tissues. If there is a lack of blood supply due to peripheral vascular disease, then you won't be able to transport healing factors and oxygen to the wound. Your body uses the oxygen to kill bacteria and heal wounds. Smoking decreases oxygen and increases carbon monoxide in the tissues while the nicotine clamps down on small blood vessels in the wound. Try to make all serious efforts at quitting smoking, getting your blood sugars under control, and exercising to increase blood flow.

Clean small wounds with soapy water, apply a double or triple antibiotic ointment and cover it with a bandage. If the wound is sustained by laceration with a dirty surface and you have not had a tetanus vaccination in more than 5 years, you may need a booster vaccination. See the chapter on tetanus. Continue to clean the wound daily with soap and reapply the ointment and bandage daily. There are wound cleansers available at the drugstore which are better than soap for daily cleaning. Try to avoid overuse of hydrogen peroxide as it may inhibit wound healing. Limit its use to initial cleaning of the dirty wound.

Persistent wounds may need the assistance of a wound care center. Physicians at these centers are experts in the use of special bandages and ointments that can assist in the healing of your wound. If you have a wound that persists despite the above care and you have risk factors for vascular disease such as age, high cholesterol, high blood pressure, or family history of heart or vascular disease, then you should have your arterial flow evaluated with an arterial Doppler ultrasound of the affected extremity

A small word about wound infections related to bites: Many significant human, dog, cat, and other animal bites become infected. Seek medical attention immediately for antibiotic therapy if you sustain any bite from an animal that pierces the skin. I have even seen infections from bites that don't pierce the skin, so watch vigilantly. The resulting skin infection can be very aggressive and can cause loss of limb. A fist fight between humans that lacerates the hand in contact with teeth is the same as a bite and requires antibiotics immediately.

It would be impossible to talk about every type of wound but it is sufficient to say that infected wounds can become serious quickly. If there is redness or drainage, seek medical care promptly. Difficult to treat wounds should be seen by both a wound care specialist and an infectious disease specialist. I have seen too many wounds treated with a combination of the free or low cost antibiotics such as cephalexin and ciprofloxacin until too late in the process to save the toe, foot, or leg. When I first started practice many years ago, a young lady enrolled in a health maintenance organization (HMO) insurance came to me after a few months of several rounds of oral ciprofloxacin. Her thumb was three times its normal size and was draining. She had not had any cultures and was told not to seek other care. She went to see a dermatologist who called our office to see the patient that day. We called her primary care physician for authorization to see the patient and were told "We told her not to go see anyone else." and were denied authorization. We sent the patient to the emergency room and started the patient on intravenous antibiotics but it was too late to save the thumb.

I could recount every one of the amazing people I have seen with some horrible wounds and each one of them has a story of how the wound progressed. Some are of their own doing, like IV drug users or trauma, and some are due to chronic illness like diabetes, but through a combination of antibiotics and wound care there can be a successful outcome. I hope through these pages I can get people to seek care sooner and become educated on how to prevent the horrible outcomes.

To recap, if there are a few actions you can do to prevent MRSA infections, they would be frequent hand washing and keeping any wounds clean and dry. Be aware of the risks of infection with chronic disease and obtain prompt medical consultation with your primary care physician, a wound care center, or an infectious disease physician. I firmly believe the specialties of wound care and infectious disease, along with vascular surgery, are limb saving specialties that work together. There are specialty clinics of sorts that are increasing in popularity called limb saving programs. These are essentially a multidisciplinary group of physicians providing care, usually at a wound care center. Even without this type of clinic you can make your own limb preservation program by seeking opinions of multiple specialists.

https://www.niaid.nih.gov/research/mrsa-methicillin-resistant-staphylococcus-aureus

Chapter 4

～

Vancomycin Resistant Enterococcus (VRE)

Enterococcus is a bacterium that is among the normal flora of the skin and gastrointestinal tract which means that it is normally found among the trillions of bacteria on our skin or in the intestines. When *Enterococcus* can become resistant to the antibiotic vancomycin, and when it does, it is called VRE (Vancomycin Resistant *Enterococcus*). There has been considerable interest in this bacterium in the last 30 years due to resistance issues. When VRE was first discovered, there were very few options for treatment of infections occurring with this bacterium. In fact, the only way to treat it was to give high doses of three antibiotics the bacterium was resistant to. After this bacterium spread within hospitals there was a call to arms to prevent such spreading. However, now we have multiple antibiotics that are effective so it has taken a backseat to other more invasive or difficult to treat bacteria such as methicillin resistant *Staphylococcus aureus* (MRSA), extended spectrum beta lactamase (ESBL) producing organisms such as *E. coli* and *Klebsiella*, and carbapenemase resistant organisms.

Colonization refers to the normal, benign, presence of bacteria in sites such as the skin, intestines, bladder, nose, or throat. *Enterococcus* is found in all of these places in healthy people without causing an infection in most cases. For example, bacteria, including *Enterococcus*, are present in the bladder in small numbers and are expelled by normal urine flow, thus keeping the bacteria population to a minimum. When a culture is obtained from the skin, wound, stool and urine the physician must always keep in mind that the bacteria found may be colonizing and not an infection, and therefore may not need to be treated. *Enterococcus* is not an inherently invasive bacterium and can be present in an open wound and not cause an infection. That is not to mean that it never causes infection, just that it lacks the qualities of a more invasive bacteria such as *Staphylococcus aureus*. For example, if the wound is deeper and closed off from the skin, the environment could be right for growth of VRE. Also, if the bacteria escape the intestines into a normally sterile environment, it could cause an infection. This happens if the intestines perforate (a hole in the intestines) or an abscess forms in the abdomen (including liver, spleen, pancreas, or kidney) or in the perianal or perirectal area. In the urine of a patient who has urinary retention or other decreased flow of urine, *Enterococcus* could also cause an infection. This is all complex information, but suffice to say it takes a severe situation for *Enterococcus* (and thus VRE) to cause an infection.

Hospitals have been surveying for this bacteria by taking samples, usually in the form of a swab, from the rectum of at risk patients and testing them for VRE. This stems from past more so than present fears of transmission in the hospital. When a patient tests positive for VRE on a surveillance culture, the patient is placed on "contact precautions", meaning workers and visitors must wear gloves and gowns to enter the room. If VRE is found on a rectal swab, that patient is deemed to be colonized with VRE and does not have an infection. If a nurse or doctor gets some of the VRE on his or her hands and walks into the room of a patient with a weakened immune system or other risk for infection, that second patient could become colonized with VRE and an infection could develop. The gowns, gloves, and diligent hand washing will help prevent this spread.

So, how does one acquire VRE? There are two main species of *Enterococcus,* and if there is one of these species present in the intestines of an individual, and they are exposed to antibiotics, there is a high likelihood that the *Enterococcus* will turn on a gene that is already present in the bacteria causing it to become vancomycin resistant. A patient could test positive on a rectal swab for VRE due to transmission from healthcare providers to that patient or because they were given an antibiotic which caused it. Since that VRE colonization (again, not infection) is no different than the usual enterococcus found in everyone's intestines, this is not so much a problem for the patient unless they have disrupted intestinal mucosa (e.g. diverticulitis, peritonitis or perforated intestines) or have a propensity to have

UTI's. It is more of a problem to the hospital that is trying to prevent the health care workers from spreading the VRE from one patient to another.

In my opinion, the need for isolation of VRE patients in hospitals is antiquated. However, there are studies regarding reduced transmission of VRE in hospitals due to institution of isolation procedures. A theoretical reason for keeping these patients in isolation would be to prevent the VRE from transferring the gene for vancomycin resistance to other bacteria. This is a moot point because there are thousands of patients with VRE colonization that are not identified. If we want to decrease this transfer, more attention could be paid to decreasing antibiotic usage as this may be far more effective.

More important than isolation in preventing spread of VRE from one patient to another is proper hand washing. The majority of patients with VRE colonization are not identified and therefore are not in isolation. Each and every time a healthcare worker enters either a hospital room or outpatient exam room and again upon exiting, he or she should wash their hands with either soap and water or an alcohol based hand sanitizer. Doctors, nurses, techs and even dietary personnel bringing your meal should be washing their hands. The reason we teach the personnel in my hospitals to wash hands consistently for every entry into a room is that even when a nurse intends to only walk into the room without touching anything, inevitably the patient asks for something as simple as adjusting a pillow. If that health care worker did not wash their hands, bacteria from their hands is now within inches from the patient's head on the pillow. Gloves should be used when handling any bodily fluid or caring for any wound or manipulating any intravenous access device.   See the chapter on hospital infections or nursing facility infections regarding hand washing.

I hear the question often, "If my husband is isolated for VRE at the hospital, shouldn't he be isolated at home?" The answer to this question lies in the level of protection that is necessary based on individual and family circumstances. If either the patient or any family member is at risk for infections, there may be some concern for spread of the bacteria. However, in most cases only "standard precautions" need to be taken. Standard precautions is a term used in hospitals indicating when one is handling bodily fluids or open wounds then gloves are to be worn.   Gowns and eye protection are also worn if fluids are likely to splash. Hand washing at home should be increased to a strict level for both the colonized person and the at-risk individual. In addition, the cleaning of personal care areas should be addressed. Diluted bleach solutions should be used frequently for bathrooms, toilets, sinks, and showers. Sheets, pillowcases and underwear should be cleaned in hot water with bleach.

If the patient or any family member has an open wound, then extra precautions should be taken. As with any wound, it should not be touched without gloves. Cleansing of the skin outside of the wound with antibacterial cleansers should be performed if directed by the surgeon or physician. Usually only special cleansers are used directly on open wounds. If a family member has a weakened immune system, such as leukemia, lymphoma, or is undergoing chemotherapy, they may be at a slightly increased risk of infection. These individuals often have intravenous ports for chemotherapy and extra care of these is necessary. Cleaning the skin around the port with chlorhexidine soap or other disinfectant as directed by your physician before accessing and after de-accessing the port may be necessary. Follow the directions of your oncologist. This is usually part of standard care of ports.

Again, hand washing is of utmost importance. Children under one year of age are also at slight risk of infection, but their immune system is usually assisted by antibodies present from their mother. Persons and family members who have frequent urinary tract infections may be at a slight risk of developing a urinary tract infection with VRE, but probably no more risk than any other bacteria and therefore should institute standard precautions and frequent hand washing.

In addition to the above, as mentioned previously, one risk of acquiring colonization with VRE is usage of certain antibiotics. Therefore, judicious use of antibiotics is always wise. Obviously your physician should direct your healthcare, so listen to his or her direction. Do not use leftover antibiotics from a previous prescription unless directed by your physician. If used as directed, there shouldn't be any left over. Use probiotics if you have no contraindication and as directed by your physician. Probiotics can ensure that your intestines contain a variety of benign bacteria that will promote colon health.

In summary, VRE, while potentially dangerous, is a weak bacteria that causes infections in certain situations. The best way to protect yourself is to use standard precautions and to assure that your health care providers (nurses, doctors, and anyone involved in your care) wash their hands before and after entering your hospital room or outpatient exam room. If a family member has VRE, you can use these same standard precautions.

For more information:

VRE. **http://www.cdc.gov/HAI/organisms/vre/vre.html**

Old information from 1995 but useful.

http://www.cdc.gov/mmwr/preview/mmwrhtml/00039349.htm

Chapter 5

~

Travel Related Infections

Picture this: You are on the vacation of a lifetime. You have finally made the trip to that exotic location and the trip does not end well. You have fever, abdominal pain, vomiting and diarrhea. Uggghhh!! This is not paradise! Let's face it, people worldwide are travelling more without researching the true risks they face. Even persons in third world countries have the means and reasons to travel to faraway places. So now, not only are Americans and Europeans travelling to third world countries and contracting unusual infections, they are not protecting themselves starting at the jet way. When I was younger and more naive, I made the mistake of eating a goat cheese sandwich while on a horseback riding excursion in Costa Rica which I paid dearly for. I was at the beginning of my Infectious Diseases training and this was the first time that I started to think about protecting myself during travel. As mentioned previously, fully 40% of travelers will develop an infection during their excursion. It is how you protect yourself that will determine whether your trip will go off without a hiccup or turn into another casualty of traveler's diarrhea ("Montezuma's revenge") or worse. To simplify, there are two things you need to avoid to protect yourself during travel: water (including uncooked food because it has come in contact with water) and insects.

It goes without saying that in less developed countries there exists less infrastructure for clean water, effective sewage and public health. We have all heard the warnings to drink bottled water in foreign countries but the warnings about clean water go far beyond that for it is not only the water you drink that can harm you, but it is the water used in cooking,

36

washing dishes, cleaning tables, and even irrigating crops that will be the unseen killer of your vacation. Sick individuals that live in these countries will be even more likely than people in the US to go to work at that quaint little roadside restaurant, use the same public facilities you will use, and not seek medical care until late in their illness. These three factors make it even more likely for you to contract illnesses from these sick people while travelling to other countries.

The most common and most written about illness contacted while travelling is Montezuma's revenge or traveler's diarrhea. There are other more serious forms of diarrhea that can occur, one of which, Typhoid fever, is very preventable with a vaccine. The diarrhea can range from watery stools to bloody stool, or there can be no diarrhea, but abdominal pain and fever the only symptoms. In addition, parasites can be ingested or absorbed through the skin. These parasites sometimes do not produce diarrhea as one would expect.

Mosquito borne illnesses stretch most of the globe in the tropical regions, including Central America, the Caribbean, South America, Africa, the Middle East, Asia, and the islands of the Pacific. Depending on the country, mosquitoes carry Yellow Fever, Dengue Fever, Chikungunya, Encephalitis viruses including Japanese Encephalitis Virus or West Nile Virus, and/or Malaria ready to inject them directly into your bloodstream. A new mosquito borne virus, Zika virus, is making its way around the globe. Zika virus causes an illness with fever, muscle aches, rash, and sometimes red eyes. It can also be sexually transmitted, making it different from these other viruses. Similar to Chikungunya and Dengue Fever, this virus will persist for a decade or longer unless we are able to provide a vaccine soon. There is a difficulty perfecting vaccines for all of these viruses due to potentially dangerous side effects and a lack of efficacy for some vaccines. These mosquito borne viruses are already making their way into the US and Europe so we need to become educated about them. Lastly, sexually transmitted diseases occur frequently during travel and will not be discussed here but can be referenced in the chapter on STDs.

Traveler's diarrhea, which has been documented in literature and in history, has had remarkable consequences throughout time for invading armies or explorers. It is safe to say that we are repeating history as the invading army of tourists succumb to these illnesses. Traveler's diarrhea usually refers to *E coli* and milder strains of *Salmonella* that cause a short duration of illness not usually requiring treatment unless there are extenuating circumstances. *E coli* has many different strains that cause varying degrees of illness. The two more virulent strains are enteroinvasive *E coli* (EIEC) and enterohemorrhagic *E coli* (EHEC). As their names imply, these strains inflict injury on the intestines by invading the mucosa and causing hemorrhage in the case of EHEC. Less severe forms of traveler's diarrhea are caused by enterotoxigenic *E* coli or ETEC.

All bacteria causing traveler's diarrhea release toxins which have varying effects, from increased secretion of water from the body into the intestines to cell damage. This water in the intestines causes the diarrhea and the loss of water from the body into the intestines causes dehydration. In the less severe forms of traveler's diarrhea (ETEC) the most severe symptom for the affected person is the diarrhea, which has been described as rice water for the almost clear fluid that results from salt and water excretion into the intestines. The greatest risk is dehydration and electrolyte abnormalities. *Vibrio cholerae*, the agent that causes cholera, is a similar example of this type of diarrhea. There are other types of bacteria that have a cholera-like toxin that mimics cholera. Hydration is the mainstay of treatment that in third world countries can be difficult causing a high infant mortality rate.

In the more severe forms of traveler's diarrhea, it is the cell damage, however, that inflicts the most damage and increases the chance of death. EHEC, *Campylobacter*, *Salmonella*, and *Shigella* are the bacteria responsible for this type of illness. Abdominal pain, fever and other symptoms predominate more so than diarrhea and for some bacteria, blood in the stool is present. It only takes ingestion of a dozen tiny bacteria of *Shigella sonnei* to cause a severe and contagious bloody diarrhea. This would be the amount on one single grain of rice. This bacteria can be spread from one person to another easily. Some bacteria such as *Salmonella typhi* invade into the bloodstream and can be deadly. There is very little if no diarrhea present, with only fever, abdominal pain, and rash as the predominant symptoms.

This is called Typhoid Fever or enteric fever and has been a public health nightmare for centuries due to its contagiousness (e.g. Typhoid Mary).

Viruses also can cause diarrheal illnesses while travelling, including the global *Norwalk* or *Norovirus, Rotavirus, Adenovirus*, and a whole host of other enteroviruses. These viruses are much more contagious than bacteria and far more common. They often require more thorough cleaning with bleach compounds and therefore easily spread in the crowded confines of a cruise ship or tropical resort. In the winter in Florida, we can't go a month without hearing of a cruise ship quarantined due to *Norovirus*, but those of you up North will not hear these stories as often so are not as familiar with it. I will mention Hepatitis A virus here because it can be spread in the same fashion. It is spread by a restaurant worker who unwittingly goes to work during the several days prior to or during his or her symptoms of illness which may be relatively unnoticeable. Hepatitis A is commonly contracted during travel to underdeveloped countries. A similar illness, Hepatitis E is particularly dangerous during travel for pregnant women.

While on vacation, it becomes entirely necessary to be more observant of the processes that are in place that could inflict injury upon you. Let's start with water and food, and then move on to the more serious vector of disease, the mosquito. Water is all around you when you travel and you hardly notice it. In America we take for granted that even the puddles in the street, while we somewhat avoid them, are relatively clean. We think nothing of stepping in a shallow pool of water as we cross the street because we have never suffered the consequences of not thinking about it. Some Americans take pride in having their children get muddy on a rainy day and there is now the popular fitness pastime of running a race through mud called a "mudder". It is this casual attitude when it comes to water that you will need to correct in order for you to get through your trip unscathed.

Water is used to clean the tables and dishes on which you eat in restaurants. In your hometown, your local health departments have the tough job of regulating restaurants and their cleanliness, which is not always the best. One of the most strictly enforced rules is the temperature of the dishwashing water which must be at least 180 degrees Fahrenheit to kill viruses and bacteria more effectively. There is no such regulation in some countries, so what workers rely on is cold, dirty dishwater in a sink for washing the dishes that come to your table. The plates are visibly clean but they are not always devoid of bacteria and viruses. Water to clean the tables and the work surfaces in the kitchen is often the same unsanitary water. Any fruit or vegetable you are served fresh may have been washed in the very same water that was used to clean the kitchen work surfaces. The same can be said for the water used to clean your hotel room, the train, the cab, the airport, the ferry, the rickshaw seats, the rental car, and the grocery store, to name just a few. The list goes on, essentially anything you touch must be scrutinized.

If you can avoid it, do so, but if you must eat from a buffet, look to see which part of the serving tray has the flame just below it. Scrape off the top portion and take the food that is at the bottom of the tray just above the flame. The key with all food is to make sure it is piping hot. Avoid roadside stands unless the food is very hot. If you toast your own toast, make it dark toast and do not use the jelly unless it comes in commercial packets. Butter may not be okay because it may not be pasteurized.

One must be always aware of the dangers of unclean water. Therefore, in addition to always drinking bottled water, make sure the bottle cap is sealed when you buy it. One way to assure that the bottled water is not just a refilled bottle of dirty parasite-infested tap water is to buy a case of bottles of water when you first arrive in country. The two layers of protection of the sealed box and the sealed cap are reassuring. Use only this bottled water for tooth brushing, or learn to brush your teeth without water. Another way to protect yourself is to drink only canned beverages or bottled sodas. You need to be observant of the condition of the top of the can for contamination as these cans can get soiled. You can sanitize it with an alcohol swab but make sure to do it thoroughly. Bottled sodas are hard to adulterate due to the carbonation, but cans are easier to visualize the seal. Bottle tops are less likely to come into contact with contaminants than are cans.

One can always boil water and it is common at tea shops for tourists to ask for boiled water. You can bring along a tea or coffee making device that will boil the water for you. Remember those small ramen noodle soup making devices you had in college? They still make them. An alternative involves sterilizing water with iodine or chlorine tablets. There are also devices that can sterilize water with filters. None of these methods is as effective as boiling. When you shower, do not ingest the water, and be careful not to wipe your mouth with the water or the towel. Use flip-flops on your feet when in the shower and, if you must be barefoot in the bathroom, put the towel down on the floor.

Using ice in your drink is also not advisable to have in your drink as it is usually made from tap water. Drink your cocktails warm and do not purchase frozen drinks. You may think they are great for that tropical vacation, but the material that exits your body later will not be pretty. It is not being impolite to turn down the glass of water at a restaurant or someone's home. "I will take a rum and coke with no ice please." Check to see how they make the Coke, out of a can or fountain, and if possible ensure there is adequate carbonation. You can ask for a shot of rum and a can of Coke so that you can prepare it correctly. When you leave the hotel, always bring along bottled water as tours and restaurants will not always have it available. Remember to buy that case of water as soon as you check in.

Again, the rule of thumb to follow: "if it is not hot when it touches your lips, do not eat it." Eat only peelable or cooked fruits and vegetables; bring your own peeler if you want to enjoy fresh peeled fruits. Bananas, apples and oranges are perfect snacks because they can be peeled. Melons could be adulterated so be aware - they are sometimes injected with unsanitary water to make them weigh more. Be aware of foods that are not completely cooked or pasteurized like they are in the US or Europe such as milk, cheeses and orange juice. Remember my goat cheese experience? Consider bringing along disposable alcohol, bleach, or ammonia-based antibacterial wipes to use in your hotel room or at your table in a restaurant. If you are concerned about the sanitation of the eating surface, order food to go, as the styrofoam packaging is possibly cleaner than the plate it could be served on or the fork you may use.

Unfortunately our "only eat food while it is hot" is not 100% foolproof, as there are toxins that could be present in cooked foods that may cause a toxin-based vomiting and diarrhea syndrome. This illness is not caused by the bacteria finding its way into your intestines, but by the toxin that was previously produced by the bacteria and currently present in the food you are eating. The toxin can survive the hot temperatures of cooking and the acid in your stomach while the bacteria cannot. An example of this is fried rice that has toxins from the bacterium *Bacillus cereus*. Staphylococcal toxins also could cause illness in cooked foods (especially mayonnaise based foods like potato salad and coleslaw) if they are left unrefrigerated for some time. Cole slaw should be a avoided anyway because it is made with uncooked cabbage. These illnesses usually have a quick onset within 30 to 90 minutes after eating the food. They are usually self-limited and require no treatment except hydration.

The time to start thinking of prevention is at least a month before you leave home. You can protect yourself from diarrheal illnesses when you travel by being prepared while packing. If you are susceptible to diarrheal illnesses or if you would risk severe illness if you did contract traveler's diarrhea you can bring along a prescription for antibiotics to start at the first sign of a significant diarrheal illness. Fill the prescription before you leave so that you are not stuck without it. Ciprofloxacin and rifaximin are common antibiotics used for this purpose. Pack iodine tablets and a tea making device (the ramen noodle cooker) for the trip just in case you cannot avoid unsanitary water. These can be bought online or in sporting goods stores with a camping section. Bring along alcohol wipes and/or bleach wipes to wipe down surfaces, making sure the alcohol drying time is at least 10 minutes, which is more than just a casual wipe. Plan where you will buy supplies such as water before you leave. Markets in some locations have provisioning websites or delivery available to your hotel.

An unproven, but potentially useful item could be a small handheld ultraviolet light device that can sterilize an exposed area with less than a two minute timeframe depending on the device. This device could sterilize a plate, silverware, a counter, or a table where you are eating. However, be aware, that it only works on surfaces and may not work for spores such as Botulism. It will not sterilize food or water and it is relatively unproven for the purposes above. I find the idea intriguing though, and would not leave home without it, for those situations where you must eat in a filthy area.

In addition, or if you do not have an antibiotic, bring chewable tablets of bismuth subsalicylate, which are available over the counter at your drug store. Proven to be just as good as antibiotics for less severe traveler's diarrhea or ETEC, this compound will bind some toxin from the bacteria and may decrease the severity of illness. Not all traveler's diarrhea needs treatment with antibiotics, so be careful what you are treating and only take antibiotics on the advice of your physician. Most traveler's diarrhea is self-limited, meaning it does not need treatment. Hydration is the most important treatment, including a low sugar, electrolyte drink. This is commonly called ORS or oral rehydration solution, and is a combination of dextrose (sugar) and salts. It can easily be made while in country using premade packets sold at many stores or markets or can be made with sugar or honey and salt. Potassium can be added if needed and is sold in some of the salt substitute products. Before taking potassium supplementation, care should be taken and a physician consulted if you already had kidney issues prior to travel. There are some recipes for this that you can get online.

There are other bacteria, viruses and parasites that may not be treated by the antibiotics mentioned above, so if you do treat yourself with antibiotics, be aware of this. *Giardia lamblia* is one of the more common parasites that you will encounter and differs from the bacteria mentioned before in that it is commonly a milder, later onset diarrhea with cramping, bloating, and a characteristic malodorous gassiness. It is usually acquired in the wilderness or from contact with someone who has had the illness. This is the illness I contracted from the goat cheese sandwich so would not have been treated with the usual antibiotics. This malady requires either tinidazole or metronidazole for 7 days. Other parasites such as *Isospora*, *Cryptosporidium*, *Microsporidium*, *Cyclospora*, and *Strongyloides* will be more difficult to diagnose and will require a physician visit. Some hotels and resorts will have English-speaking physicians with access to relatively sophisticated testing at your request.

Never walk barefoot in any area of a foreign country including your hotel room. Parasites can enter the skin of your feet and travel to different areas of your body. One such parasite is *Strongyloides stercoralis*. Travelling from your feet to your lungs, it is then coughed up and swallowed where it enters your intestines, invades the mucosa, then travels again to your lungs, creating a chronic cycle of mild cough that on chest x ray seems like a migratory pneumonia. Also present in the soil and water are parasites such as *Schistosoma*, bacteria such as *Leptospira* and *Actinomy-*

ces, and invasive molds such as *Mucor*. *Leptospira* causes pneumonia with a possible jaundice and is not treated with the usual antibiotics. *Actinomyces* and *Mucor* can cause skin infections in diabetic and liver failure patients.

Now that we have avoided unsanitary water, we need to rid ourselves of the pesky bugs. There are many genera and species of mosquitoes, but only one genus (*Anopheles*) with about 100 species of mosquitoes can transmit malaria. This genus also transmits multiple other diseases in tropical and subtropical areas around the world. The *Aedes* genus is responsible for transmitting the viruses associated with Dengue fever, Chikungunya fever, Zika virus, Yellow Fever, and other encephalitis viruses. This genus is present in the US in low numbers but has, for the most part, been controlled well since the yellow fever outbreaks of the 1960's. *Aedes* mosquitoes proliferate in tropical zones especially in underdeveloped countries. Other genera of mosquitoes such as *Culex* spread encephalitis (such as West Nile Virus) throughout the world including the US.

Malaria has been prevalent for centuries and kills more people in the world than any other infectious disease. It is currently present in Africa, Asia, the Pacific Islands, Central and South America, Dominican Republic and Haiti. Approximately 300 million people contract malaria and 1 million people die every year from it. Malaria was described in Chinese medical writings and hieroglyphic writings in the tombs of Egypt. It killed Amerigo Vespucci and many other explorers of the 16th to 19th centuries. It also spread to the temperate zones of Europe and the Americas before being eradicated from these temperate zones in the 1940s. This parasite infects its host's red blood cells and causes an illness marked by fever, muscle aches, dark urine, jaundice (yellowing of the skin or eyes) and confusion. The amount of confusion depends on the species, as this symptom will predominate in patients infected with *Plasmodium falciparum*, often called cerebral malaria due to the hallmark delirium. This is the most deadly form of malaria. There are three other species of malaria in humans: *Plasmodium malariae*, *Plasmodium vivax*, and *Plasmodium ovale*. The parasites of *P. vivax* and *ovale* can hide in the liver for up to 4 weeks and emerge again to cause fever if treatment (or preventive medication) is not continued long enough.

Treatments for malaria have been in existence for a few thousand years from Chinese medicine writings. They used herbs from the qinghao plant that appear to have had the chemical artemisinin which is in some modern medications that are now becoming the most effective for malaria. Another older medication, quinine, was also thought to have helped eradicate the disease in the developed world. Malarone, quinine, and artemisinin are often used to treat patients. These medications also prevent the disease if taken continuously during exposure. It is highly recommended to take malaria prevention or prophylaxis medications while travelling to malaria-prone areas, including Central and South America, Africa, Asia, the Pacific Islands, Haiti and Dominican Republic. There are four main medications to take to prevent malaria, chloroquine, mefloquine, doxycycline, and atovaquone/proguanil. Central America, Haiti, and the Middle East are the only areas where it is recommended to take chloroquine. Mefloquine may have significant neurologic side effects and is often not used but is cheap. Doxycycline has few side effects, except some gastro intestinal side effects and the possibility of a sun exposure induced rash. Atovaquoe/proguanil is often the preferred prevention medication for travelers from the US and has few side effects but is expensive. Your travel physician will have more information for you to choose the appropriate medication.

It is important to take the medications as directed. All of these medications need to be taken for a few days to a week prior to arrival at the destination and for a week to four weeks following return home, depending on the medication. The extra time is needed to treat the malaria parasites that will emerge from their hiding place in your liver if not treated. Discuss with your doctor or travel clinic which medication is best for you. Your life could depend on it. Remain vigilant to avoid mosquitoes during your entire trip because it is not just malaria you are trying to avoid. I remember a trip to Delhi, India where inside the airport there were more mosquitoes than the outer villages of Delhi. It was the only time I did not have DEET on. Needlessly to say, I was swatting at mosquitoes for 2 hours at my gate, hoping to avoid dengue or chikungunya virus infections. I had not missed any doses of malarone so I was not so worried about malaria.

I have heard many anecdotes of people in positions of authority who have told others that they do not need to take preventive medications for malaria. These include employers of sales people travelling overseas and clergy supervising missionaries going to Africa. One such clergy member told an employee of a nearby hospital that when she went on a mission to Africa that she didn't need to take malaria prophylaxis. Luckily she listened to me, because that pastor became so ill he had to be carried by bush people for 20 miles to a local hospital and had cardiac arrest upon his arrival there.

I have witnessed patients returning from a six month trip to Africa who had skipped just a few doses of malaria prophylaxis within a week prior to returning home that became very ill with malaria after they returned. One such patient who skipped a few doses was a public health student and I swear she skipped some doses just to say she had contracted malaria. She arrived in the states just in time to start the fever and presented saying, "I have malaria." I have also heard people being told by others, probably a myth left over from the days when mefloquine was a popular choice, that the drug is worse than the disease. Please remember that malaria is the number one killer out of all infections worldwide when you are listening to these uninformed people.

Yellow fever is a vaccine preventable disease carried by the *Aedes* mosquitoes mainly in Africa and South America. The CDC's book on travel and vaccination recommendations is called the Yellow Book and your vaccination card is yellow and the quarantine flag for shipping and customs is yellow because of this disease. Many countries that have no yellow fever require the vaccine for entry because they do not want any new cases brought in from outside the country. It is highly recommended and required to receive the vaccine to enter countries with yellow fever present. While highly effective, the vaccine is not 100% effective and there are other diseases transmitted by mosquitoes; therefore, it is still necessary to avoid mosquitoes using the following measures.

Other mosquito borne illnesses such as Zika virus, Chikungunya Fever, Dengue Fever, West Nile Fever and other encephalitis viruses have no vaccine, preventive medication, or current treatment. Therefore, mosquito avoidance is the mainstay of prevention and one needs to take the necessary precautions to prevent these potentially fatal illnesses. We have seen a steady number of returning travelers with Dengue and an explosion of people with Chikungunya due to the recent arrival and rapid spread of Chikungunya through the Caribbean and Central and South America in

2013. The newest of these related viruses is Zika virus which arrived in South and Central America in 2015 and spread to the US in 2016. These illnesses are also present in Asia and Africa where Chikungunya, Dengue, and Zika virus originated, spreading later to the Western Hemisphere. The only other vaccine for a mosquito-borne virus for general use is the Japanese encephalitis virus vaccine which is recommended for travelers to certain areas of Asia during some seasons. Usually only infectious disease physicians and travel clinics will be aware of its use. Another virus originating from South America, Mayaro virus, could be the next candidate to spread, as it has recently been found in a patient in Haiti.

What is certain over the past 40 years is that nothing spreads faster across most of the world than a mosquito-borne virus. It seems we have just become accustomed to diagnosing one virus when the next one is discovered. A special mention here about Zika virus because it is not only spread by the mosquito bite. Previous mosquito borne viruses have a limit of how far they can be spread geographically by the location of the mosquito and the fact the mosquito cannot effectively reproduce when the temperature is below 40 to 50 degrees Fahrenheit. However, if a virus can be spread sexually in addition to via the mosquito, there could be further penetration of the virus among populations that would not normally be at risk.

There is significant evidence that the Zika virus can be transmitted from one person to another sexually; however, it is not known how efficiently it is spread in this manner. The significance of this is tremendous, because of the ramifications of the Zika virus infection that is associated with a birth defect in pregnant women called microcephaly. We are just starting to be aware of other major developmental issues that will occur in the fetus of a pregnant woman infected with Zika virus that may not be known for several years. The theory is that, similar to the childhood developmental abnormalities seen with cytomegalovirus, there could be similar issues seen years after pregnancy with Zika virus. There are recommendations for pregnant women to take certain precautions with travel and mosquito exposure in addition to sexual exposures to men who have travelled to areas of Zika virus transmission. The latest recommendations can be found on the CDC website. **http://www.cdc.gov/zika/**

Chikungunya and Zika viruses may have spread so rapidly because they have acquired the ability to reproduce readily in *Aedes aegypti* and a special species called *Aedes albopictus* which is also called the Asian tiger mosquito. This mosquito is widespread in all continents including North America. What is different about this mosquito is that it bites humans during the daytime and lives closer to human dwellings. In addition, it bites multiple times and bites multiple people in the same blood meal so it can spread these two viruses more rapidly. Other mosquitoes only bite one person, so would only be able to spread a virus to one person per day. In addition, their bites can be almost imperceptible, allowing them to spread the virus without detection.

The symptoms of Zika virus, Chikungunya, Dengue and a few other mosquito borne viruses are similar and include muscle and joint pain, fever, headache, red eyes and a rash. Dengue virus has a potentially fatal hemorrhagic or bleeding symptom that uncommonly occurs. For this reason, non-steroidal anti-inflammatory medications like ibuprofen and aspirin are avoided in cases of dengue. If you return from an area with these viruses and have these symptoms it may be wise to consult the CDC website above for current recommendations on mosquito avoidance and sexual abstinence. Because of the similarities among these viral illnesses, in order to be accurately diagnosed, one would need to be tested for all of three of the viruses.

Avoiding mosquitos entirely in tropical countries is difficult to accomplish because all it takes is a small amount of skin exposure for one to land and start feeding. It is recommended that you cover as much of the skin as possible and couple this with application of a mosquito repellant to the skin and clothes. The repellant should have DEET with at least 25% concentration. This concentration is found in some of the more advanced formulas, sometimes referred to as "Deep Woods" or other names. The concentration is usually found in the ingredients label. There are 100% DEET formulations that can be used also, but do not offer better protection than 25% formulations, but they do last longer. In one study, a 4.75% DEET concentration protected for only a little more than an hour, while 23.8% DEET protected for over 5 hours. It is unclear how much longer 100% DEET formulations will last, but they may be more toxic to your body or damaging to the fabric in your clothes.

There are also effective area sprays and coils that you can spray in a room or wear attached to your clothing, but these need to be coupled with a repellant applied to the skin. Products such as wrist bands or coils do not work alone. Clothing can be treated with permethrin or it can be bought already pretreated with permethrin. If sleeping in a less secure (inadequately screened or non-air conditioned) environment, use a permethrin treated bed net. Be aware that sunscreens can inactivate insect repellants therefore one must apply the sunscreen first, let it dry, and then apply the mosquito repellant. Alternatively, one can buy a combination product called Sunsect that has been used by the military and is available commercially. These can be found at sporting and outdoors and camping stores. See the CDC's page referenced at the end of this chapter regarding these precautions.

In addition to these illnesses there are other water borne and insect borne illnesses that you need to be aware of. In Africa, the vector (the organism that spreads the disease) for African sleeping sickness or *Trypanosoma brucei* is the tsetse fly. There are multiple bacteria in a class called rickettsia that are spread by body louse, mites and other insects. The filarial parasites Wuchereria and Loa Loa are best prevented by avoiding mosquitoes and deerflies, respectively. Small flat worms called flukes, which cause liver and lung disease in humans, are best avoided by not eating their hosts: snails, fish, crustaceans and water chestnuts in foreign countries. In Central and South America, Chagas disease or *Trypanosoma cruzi* is caused by the bite of the triatomine bug (kissing bug). It lives near houses, especially in rural areas. It is a leading cause of congestive heart failure in South America. Due to immigration, it is estimated that 300,000 people in the US have this parasite in their bodies. However, it cannot be spread in the US because the kissing bug does not live here.

Ebola and other hemorrhagic viruses are present in Central Africa in countries such as Congo, Democratic Republic of Congo, Uganda, Sierra Leone, Guinea, Liberia, Nigeria, Sudan, Kenya, and Angola, and also in the Philippines. The reservoir (an animal that harbors the virus without illness) for Marburg and Ebola is the African fruit bat. Primates (including humans) and other animals then become infected through direct contact with or ingestion of a fruit that has been partially eaten by the fruit bat or an infected bat or other animal. Many cases of illnesses in humans are from contact with a patient while performing medical care or during missions. In general, it is highly unusual for other travelers to become stricken with these viruses. Fortunately, the aid agencies supplying aid and medical missions to these countries have extensive experience protecting their workers. There are other hemorrhagic viruses associated with rodents around the world including the US. Please refer to the chapter on Ebola.

Bedbugs are also becoming increasingly more common not only in underdeveloped countries but now also in developed countries. They are small, flat and reddish-brown bugs. Consider looking for them at all hotel rooms upon entry; you should inspect the underside of mattresses and box springs for signs of infestation. The tell-tale sign is a small waxy area with a small bug (about a quarter of an inch or 5mm) under the mattress or box spring or inside the frame of the bed. Sometimes the only sign may be a spot of blood on the sheet leading down to the side of the mattress. Keep your suitcase off the floor and keep the lid closed. If you see any signs of bedbugs you should seek alternate lodging.

Lastly, tuberculosis (TB) is very common in many third world countries and therefore it is recommended that if you are travelling extensively among indigenous populations or performing any medical or mission work abroad that you receive a PPD (purified protein derivative) test or a blood test to evaluate for exposure to tuberculosis periodically. If you are exposed to tuberculosis unknowingly, you could develop active tuberculosis possibly many years later if you are not treated. The treatment for the exposure (called latent tuberculosis infection) is much less burdensome on you than the treatment and isolation that you will need if you contract active tuberculosis.

When you are exposed to a person with active tuberculosis, he or she coughs bacteria into the air and since, unlike other bacterium, it can float in the air, it can enter your lungs. Once it enters your lungs, your body may kill it or it may simply inactivate the live bacteria by walling it off into something called a granuloma which is microscopic and cannot be seen on X rays. From approximately a few days to a few weeks later, if you are tested with a TB skin test (when using a skin testing procedure using PPD (purified protein derivative) injected into the top layer of the skin), the test will turn positive. In addition, you will test positive on a blood test for tuberculosis. At any point in your lifetime, from years to decades later, that bacterium can break out from that shell (the granuloma) and cause a symptomatic contagious cough and pneumonia called active tuberculosis. After a positive test, 10% of persons with a normal immune system will be stricken with active TB over their lifetime of active tuberculosis. Approximately half of these will occur in the first two years and the remaining half at any point during the rest of life. People with declining immune systems due to increasing age or use of specific medications are more vulnerable. See the chapter on tuberculosis for more information.

So now you have all the tools for protecting yourself. Avoid any and all water that is not bottled. Do not swim in fresh water or walk barefoot. Buy a case of bottled water at the beginning of your trip and drink canned or bottled beverages when you can. The only foods you should eat are those that are hot when they touch your lips. Avoid mosquitoes and other insects and take malaria prophylaxis if indicated. For every country you travel to, visit the webpage for that country on the Centers for Disease Control travel website also called the Yellow Book after Yellow Fever. Go to www.cdc.gov and navigate to the Travelers page, and click on Destinations. Follow the advice there at the minimum but I highly recommend that you go to a Travel Clinic.

There are reputable travel clinic in many areas for advice. They can give you preventive medications and vaccines that could save your life. Ask your doctor for advice and do not rely on your cousin, your pastor, your Aunt Mildred, or your coworker for medical advice because those people won't have to suffer the consequences of the bad advice

For more information:

http://www.cdc.gov/travel

http://www.nejm.org/doi/full/10.1056/NEJMoa011699#t=article

List of Travel Clinics:

http://www.istm.org/AF_CstmClinicDirectory.asp

http://www.astmh.org/for-astmh-members/clinical-consultants-directory

Chapter 6

$\sim$

Prevention of Post-Surgical Infections and Wound Infections

I first met her in the office a few weeks after her C-section. Instead of enjoying her time with her newborn baby, she was dealing with a draining wound that was not responding to the usual antibiotics given by her obstetrician. Suspicious of a methicillin resistant *Staphylococcus aureus* (MRSA) wound infection, I placed her on some antibiotics that would treat this bacteria and obtained cultures that confirmed my suspicion. After two more weeks of antibiotics and wound care, she finally had a good outcome. This is just a mild example of a post-surgical wound infection. I can recount many more significant infections resulting in worse outcomes. Just a few weeks prior to publishing this book, a colleague's father had a severe infection following a very complicated pancreatic surgery called a Whipple procedure. Unfortunately, he perished from this infection at a nearby hospital. While these mild and severe cases are expected complications of surgery, hopefully the rate of these infections is low enough that a minimal number of patients have to go through these experiences. The importance of prevention and good surgical care revolves around avoiding any complication. In addition, early recognition and appropriate treatment of the complicating infection is just as important.

The discussion about complications your surgeon has with you regarding your potential surgery includes the risk of death, dismemberment, blood clots and infection. The risks are sometimes glossed over and unfortunately at times not even discussed or the discussion is made through a pre-printed brochure. The good surgeons have an open, verbal discussion with the patient about risks and benefits. The odds of infection depend on patient factors (obesity, diabetes, compliance and smoking), the complexity and location of the surgery, the surgeon, and the quality of the healthcare facility where the surgery will occur. These important points need to be discussed with the patient. The dangers are usually mentioned in the body of the consent for the procedure that the patient signs. Whatever your knowledge of the risk, you will need to learn some vital information prior to your surgery that will reduce your risk.

The rate of surgical skin infection (SSI) ranges from as low as 0.5% to as high as 8-20%. Minimally invasive surgeries such as laparoscopic and laser surgeries have infection rates on the lower end of the scale from 0.5% to 2%. Higher risk surgeries, including vascular surgeries and orthopedic surgeries are around 2-3% and emergent and so-called dirty surgeries have even higher risk. Dirty surgeries include open fracture (meaning the bone exits the skin) surgeries and abdominal surgeries where there is spillage of intestinal contents. Once there is an SSI, the risk of mortality is approximately 3% and you are between 2 and 5 times more likely to die if you have an SSI than if you do not. The stakes are high and you need to be vigilant to protect yourself.

Surgical infections are most likely to occur from the moment of the incision to approximately 24 to 48 hours after. Sometimes the wound edges are not completely adhered to each other and when this occurs the timeframe of risk can be extended. In most cases, the surgeon does not introduce the bacteria causing the infection. Often the bacteria are already present on the nearby skin or inside the patient, including the intestines as mentioned above. The offending bacteria could be introduced after surgery as bacteria migrate from outside areas to the wound. The bacteria could also be introduced into the area during dressing changes.

The bacteria that predominate in these infections are *Staphylococcus*, *Streptococcus*, and intestinal bacteria such as *E coli*. If the surgery is in the lower extremities or abdominal area, the likelihood of these difficult to treat intestinal bacteria causing an infection is slightly increased. This is due to the proximity to the groin area where these bacteria are at highest concentrations on the skin. However, even in this area of the body, staph and strep predominate.

Risk factors that predispose patients to surgical site infections include age, obesity, smoking, peripheral vascular disease, and diabetes. Older age carries with it multiple components such as decreased immune function, diminished heart function and peripheral vascular disease. The skin is also more fragile and thin in elderly individuals. In obese patients there are multiple skin folds and additional pressure causes separation of wound edges, allowing bacteria to invade. Imagine the risk of puncture of an under filled water balloon versus an overfilled one. The stretched skin has a higher likelihood of the wound edges coming apart, allowing bacteria to invade. In addition, the skin folds harbor bacteria in higher concentrations and types of bacteria that would not normally be on that particular area of skin.

Nicotine from smoking clamps down on small blood vessels in wound edges, thus retarding wound healing. Carbon dioxide and carbon monoxide present in the blood from smoking diminishes the killing power of neutrophil white blood cells (the bacterial killer cells), compounding the risk of smoking. Peripheral vascular disease inhibits wound healing especially in the extremities owing to blockage of blood vessels, which in turn causes low oxygen levels in the tissues, lower amounts of healing factors and diminished ability for infection fighting cells to get to the area of the wound. The high blood sugar of diabetes also poisons neutrophils and diminishes blood flow. The risk of infection of a diabetic patient is approximately double that of a non-diabetic. Blood sugar levels around the time of surgery are often erratic due to stress and other factors.

Apart from the characteristics of the patient, the factors of the hospital or surgical center are equally important. In general, hospitals have more staff to implement and monitor infection control practices than surgical centers. Some surgical centers do not have adequate policies in place to prevent infections; therefore you will see a more disorganized effort to control infections. Hospitals are not perfect either. It behooves all patients having surgery to monitor the infection control practices all of the nurses and doctors use during their stay. Infection prevention requires a team effort and the more people involved and included in that effort the better. There is not much data regarding the risk of infection in surgical centers, so you may not be able to research the risk for yourself.

It doesn't stop there, though. The unfortunate outcomes from infection are more likely to occur if infection is not recognized early enough, especially in hospitalized patients. There are multiple studies assessing what factors increase the mortality rate at high mortality hospitals. It is well known that a small amount of excess mortality has to do with the complexity of cases at larger, tertiary referral centers. A tertiary referral center is usually a larger hospital that has more services and therefore smaller hospitals refer more complex patients to them. It would be expected that these hospitals would have higher complication rates and higher mortality. However, this is not always the case.

The element of care that does matter most is a term called failure to resuscitate. A major component of this is early recognition of complications after surgery including infection. If infection (or any complication for that matter) is not recognized early and treated adequately, there will potentially be a poor outcome including death. Usually larger hospitals with more resources are better at doing this and smaller hospitals or other hospitals that do not have the resources to have dedicated staff and policies to spot complications are worse. Teaching hospitals have younger, less experienced physicians but these training doctors are usually more thorough and more attentive to newer technologies and newer processes to prevent infections.

So what can you do to prevent infection? First let's start with inspection of the facility and then we will discuss what you can do for yourself to prevent infection. The inspection starts prior to the anticipated day of surgery and does not stop until long after you are discharged from the facility. You should use your family members to help because there will be some time when you will be unconscious or groggy from anesthesia or pain medications. It is not just the personnel that you are scrutinizing. This is about empowerment for you to prevent errors in your care. Aside from the operating room and recovery room, you should never be without a family member from the minutes prior to surgery to the days after recovery. They will be your eyes and your advocate while you are not able to.

Research facilities using Medicare's Hospital Compare website. It can be found at **http://www.medicare.gov/hospitalcompare/search. html** and can be used to compare infection rates and policies at hospitals.

One important rate is the rate of influenza vaccination of staff, which has been associated with lower mortality at hospitals. A higher rate of influenza vaccination of staff could imply a more educated staff and a proactive, patient-centered experience where the patients are more important than staff trying to avoid vaccinations. Look under Timely and Effective Care Tab with the subheading Preventive Care. Then look at the Complications Tab and the Readmissions Tab. These can be misleading but are a good start to your research.

When monitoring staff, the biggest item to look for is handwashing. There are two methods that should be used, alcohol foam or gel and soap and water. Alcohol based sanitizers have been introduced because of the horrific rates of handwashing among healthcare personnel with soap and water. Even with this introduction, however, surveillance studies show that certainly less than 50% of personnel wash their hands in between encounters with patients. This is absolutely the antithesis of patient centered care as every healthcare provider needs to be thinking about patient safety at all times. Usually physicians are worse at hand washing than nurses who are worse than patient care techs. Surprisingly, the best compliance with handwashing in one study was the dietary personnel.

Actually this is probably not so surprising. In a restaurant or in the hospital kitchen, if you do not wash your hands there are consequences such as loss of a job. In healthcare there is little accountability. Hospitals do their own surveillance, but it is usually the case of the fox guarding the henhouse. A quality control nurse or charge nurse (who is known to everyone on the floor) is watching his or her own employees who are his or her friends. I have found hospitals reporting 90% and higher compliance and this is not likely to be true based on my own observations. The best secret shopper personnel I have found have been the dietary personnel for, again, obvious reasons.

Hand washing is the the single most important indicator of your quality care and needs to foremost in your mind for observation. Ask the nurse to give you an extra container of alcohol foam and place it in a conspicuous place like the tray table. This will make it easier for you to break the ice and ask that forgetful nurse or doctor to wash their hands. It will also allow you to wash your own hands periodically. If this is not possible, buy your own alcohol gel dispenser and bring it with you.

The nurses taking care of you should be washing their hands before and after doing anything in your room. Observe everything that the nurse or doctor does. If handling a syringe, IV, or a wound, gloves should always be worn. The cleanliness of the treatment areas should be a clue as to the quality of care given. How hurried are the nurses and providers? When placing a foley catheter or inserting an IV, do they throw unused items onto the bed while performing their function? How meticulous are they with their job? How do they handle medications? When vials of medications are opened, the tops should be cleaned with an alcohol swab prior to inserting the needle.

The correct choice of perioperative antibiotics and the correct timing of them is something that was an issue in the past, but data has been reported to the Joint Commision on Accreditation of Healthcare Organizations that largely indicates hospitals have taken care of this common error. However, this past error has been replaced by the following error. If you weigh greater than 100 kg or 220 pounds you may need a larger dose of antibiotics within 30 minutes prior to incision and many surgeons do not think of this change. In addition, surgeries that last longer than 6 hours will require a second dose of the antibiotic depending on which antibiotic is used.

The surgical scrub, which is the solution the nurses use to clean the surgical area prior to incision, can be an issue. There are three possibilities: chlorhexidine, betadine, and povidone iodine. Chlorhexidine will generally be clear, betadine will turn the skin brown, and povidone iodine will turn it yellow. Povidone and chlorhexidine also usually have alcohol in them so they need to be put on wet and allowed to dry by themselves without wiping. There is data to show that betadine is inferior to the other two products, and perhaps some data to show that chlorhexidine is superior to povidone. However, I see many surgeries in outpatient settings using betadine prep. Areas like the vaginal area and neurosurgery incision sites should not have chlorhexidine exposed to them but this is only theoretical due to the alcohol present in the chlorhexidine that could dry the tissue.

Check to see what prep is used because it should be povidone or chlorhexidine.

Now let's talk about what you can do for yourself. This is 50% of the battle. First and foremost, is your own scrub. For two decades it has been known that a preoperative bath with 2% chlorhexidine soap will reduce postoperative infections up to 50%. However it has only been commonplace to recommend it in cardiac and orthopedic procedures for the past 5-10 years. More often than not, it is not mentioned or buried in a two page tiny print preoperative instructions pamphlet. Ideally, a head to toe chlorhexidine bath should take place five nights in a row prior to surgery as this is more effective than only one day, but you should at least do one bath if you do not do five. There is significant data supporting the importance of testing you for *Staph aureus* colonization and treatment with a nasal ointment called mupirocin if the test is positive. There is some preliminary data to suggest that povidone iodine nasal ointment may be better than mupirocin. This can be obtained either by prescription or over the counter at all drug stores. The one approved for nasal use is made by 3M. Mupirocin is available only by prescription.

Obese patients and smokers are at higher risk for post-surgical infections. As mentioned above, diabetic patients have about double the infection risk of persons without diabetes. Any elective surgery should be prepared for with weight loss, smoking cessation, and glucose control. If you are over a BMI of 30 you should consider weight loss strategies prescribed by your doctor to lose weight. If you are still overweight when you have surgery, extra precautions for prevention of wound infections could involve extra-stringent hygiene, added care to prevent stretching the wound edges, and the chlorhexidine baths for 5 days prior to surgery as above. Smoking cessation is a must, even if it is for only a few days prior to surgery and during the wound healing time frame of at least 48 hours after surgery. That small amount of time should be enough to get the nicotine out of your system and cut down on the amount of carbon monoxide in your blood. Diabetic patients and those that have been told they have "borderline" diabetes should watch their carbohydrate intake and keep blood sugar levels under strict control.

It would seem this paragraph would be obvious to most, but I see, on a daily basis, otherwise intelligent people taking their dressing off and pointing to and touching an area of their wound with their bare hands. I realize that the average person who has bought this book likely already has some good habits and is not going to make this error. I need not say to you how many bacteria are on your hand and that those bacteria are staph aureus or strep species, the culprits of many wound infections. For anyone touching the wound, dressing, or the surrounding skin, gloves need to be worn at all times and handwashing is essential both before putting the gloves on and after removing them

The wound care that you perform on the wound will vary from surgery to surgery. However there are some basic tenets of post-surgical wound care. First, only clean with a bona fide wound cleanser if directed by your surgeon or physician. They can be obtained at your local drug store. Unless instructed by your doctor, do not use hydrogen peroxide on your wound for an extended period of time. Hydrogen peroxide can prevent the growth of new skin cells on the surface of the wound. There are limited circumstances when it is useful, though, so listen to your doctor. Keeping the bacterial numbers low on the surface of the wound is important for wound healing. The wound cleanser should suffice. You may be told to use a double or triple antibiotic ointment. Between 5 and 20% of people react to the neomycin portion of the triple antibiotic. If you get some irritation in the area of application, consult your doctor about switching to the double antibiotic or straight bacitracin. No matter what dressing is used, make sure that the area you are using for dressing changes is clean. Only use individually wrapped gauze. Paper tape may be better than first aid tape because it is less likely to cause skin tears.

At all cost do not make the same mistake that I see at least once or twice per year. Do NOT let your pet lick or get close to your wound. No, really! This happens.

If you have swelling of the legs (also called edema) and have a surgical wound there, you are at higher risk for infection. First, the edema is like the water in a sponge that leaks out due to gravity. That fluid will leak out of the wound which we commonly refer to as weeping. When it leaks, it carries with it the materials and cells your body is trying to lay down in the bed of the wound for healing. In addition, if there is significant edema, that extra space of tissue has poor blood supply and has very little immune system support. Make every effort to control edema, including by the simple means of leg elevation. To accomplish this, prop the leg up above the level of the heart. There are other methods that you should ask your doctor about. This includes ace bandages and the even tighter elastic bandage that self-adheres, but do not use these on an area of a surgical wound without consulting your doctor. The extra pressure may help to minimize the local edema at the wound and thus also minimize the weeping. A more absorbent dressing may be necessary to wick away the drainage so that it doesn't macerate the wound turning it white like your skin after being in the pool for too long. This white macerated skin does not heal well, therefore minimizing the wetness of the area will help prevent infection.

If you have an implanted artificial joint or an artificial heart valve, this will require special attention to prevent infections for years after surgery. For artificial joints, you will need to take preventive antibiotics each time you have dental work for the first year after surgery. Ask your dentist or your orthopedist for more information. For artificial heart valves, this need for preventive antibiotics will extend for the life of the heart valve. You may also need preventive antibiotics for other procedures such as colonoscopies if there is a biopsy. The American Heart Association publishes guidelines at **http://circ.ahajournals.org/content/116/15/1736. full?sid=c7499903-15aa-48a8-bde0-a839337fd702**

My suggestion is, at first sight of any problem with your wound, make an urgent appointment with both your surgeon and your primary care doctor. Then, immediately after these appointment make an appointment at a wound care center. These centers have physicians specially trained in wound care and have proven positive results. A consultation with a wound care center results in a 50% better likelihood of a favorable outcome and less likelihood of wound complication or amputation. These physicians are able to spend more time concentrating on the wound care and will be more likely to order the correct diagnostic studies to improve your chances of wound healing.

So, by all means, the tools to prevent that infection are in your hands. Take the bull by the horns and don't let the system that is not perfect let you down. Look to all of your health care providers for information about your wound and your particular situation. Make them perform to their abilities and responsibilities and a good outcome will be yours. Some of your family and friends will have information for you and half of it will be incorrect. There is an old adage in medical school that half of what your teachers teach you is incorrect. The only thing you have to figure out is which half is correct and which half is incorrect. Do your homework and decide which half is best for you.

More Information:

https://www.medicare.gov/hospitalcompare/search.html

http://www.cdc.gov/HAI/ssi/ssi.html

Surgical Site Infections: epidemiology, microbiology, and prevention. Journal of Hospital Infection. 2008; 70(S2):3-10. http://www.ncbi..nlm.nih.gov/pubmed/19022115

Paul J. Kim, Karen K. Evans, John S. Steinberg, Mark E. Pollard, Christopher E. Attinger, Critical elements to building an effective wound care center, Journal of Vascular Surgery, Volume 57, Issue 6, June 2013. http://www.ncbi.nlm.nih.gov/pubmed/23402873

A New Concept of a Multidisciplinary Wound Healing Center and a National Expert Function of Wound Healing. Finn Gottrup, MD, DMSc; Per Holstein, MD, DMSc; Bo Jørgensen, MD; Michael Lohmann, MD; Tonny Karlsmar, MD, DMSc. Arch Surg. 2001;136(7):765-772.

Chapter 7

~

Diabetic infections

There are approximately 30 million persons with diabetes mellitus in the United States or almost 10% of the population. There are also 1.5 million new cases of diabetes every year. This disorder of sugar metabolism has two types: Type I, which is often acquired in childhood or young adulthood and requires insulin, and Type II, which often begins in later adulthood and is associated with obesity. Approximately one third or 8 million Type II diabetics do not know they have diabetes. By the time Type II diabetes is diagnosed, it has been affecting the individual for 10 years or more. Therefore the damage that comes with diabetes has already had a head start. The increased blood sugar is often associated with excessive thirst, increased urination and fatigue, which are vague symptoms that many non-diabetics exhibit.

It is very common for me to see a patient with type II diabetes and a serious life or limb threatening infection. Diabetes can be a very manageable disease but it can also be a devastating disease if one of the many complications arise. Persons with diabetes mellitus are at risk for a multitude of infections for many reasons, including a weakened immune system, peripheral neuropathy (nerve damage usually in the legs), diminished healing factors, reduced kidney function, and altered blood flow. Skin infections, bone infections, pneumonia, urinary tract infections, and blood stream infections occur with increased frequency in these individuals.

Of the infections, the most common and devastating are diabetic foot infections. Wounds can develop on the feet due to peripheral neuropathy, the decreased sensation caused by high blood sugars over time. The constant bathing of nerves in high blood sugars poisons the nerves and the longest nerves become unresponsive to stimuli. This is manifested by numbness and burning sensations. These patients are not aware of physical overuse, and they place too much pressure on the wrong parts of their feet. A small pebble or other object could be in their shoe and they don't feel it. For either of these reasons, a callus forms, followed by a wound. In fact, a callus is nothing more than a wound with porous, ineffective skin covering it. Our feet are exposed to many bacteria in our shoes (such as *Streptococcus and Pseudomonas*) which can invade into the body when given the opportunity. A callus gives these bacteria just such an opportunity. It is a huge mistake to think a callus is normal skin. Diabetics should treat these calluses the same as open wounds.

Diabetics' high blood sugars injures their white blood cells, preventing them from accessing the wound to prevent or fight infections. These high blood sugars also alter small blood vessels causing local lack of blood flow, which further impedes wound healing and infection fighting. This is especially true when coupled with smoking, which further clamps down on local blood vessels and harms infection fighting cells, thus creating ideal conditions for an uncontrolled infection. Indeed, with the combination described above, diabetic foot infections can invade deeply and quickly to destroy deep tissues, such as bone or muscle or tendons.

Peripheral vascular disease plagues many diabetic patients. This is a more permanent blockage of the arteries than that described in the previous paragraph. Patients with diabetes often have cholesterol problems in the form of high triglycerides and this can lead to the cholesterol lining the arteries of the body, including the heart and the lower legs. The lack of blood flow that results also can be devastating to the wound healing system. Higher blood sugars also may destabilize plaque in the arteries of the legs thus worsening blood flow. Strict control of cholesterol and diabetes could minimally reverse this, but usually it requires surgical intervention to correct.

If diabetic patients take a proactive stance, especially regarding weight loss, smoking, tight blood sugar control, and visiting a podiatrist regularly, they can enjoy years of additional quality of life that many diabetic patients lose. Education on the disease process and weight loss is the cornerstone of success. This education often requires more than just visiting your primary care physician. Diabetic nurse educators will be your doorway to regaining that quality of life. And may I say again that it will require significant weight loss!! Do some research on a plant based diet, as I had a podiatrist friend who probably saved his own life by switching to a plant based diet that resulted in significant weight loss. Before we talk about the positives, let's talk about mistakes to avoid.

I recently treated a patient in this very typical diabetic patient scenario. A month prior he had gone to an amusement park where he walked all day in what seemed to be adequate shoes for a diabetic. A few days later, he developed a small blister in an area right beside a callous on the bottom of his big toe. When the area turned red, he was placed on antibiotics by his primary care physician. Initially, it improved. Unfortunately after finishing his antibiotics he had marked worsening with purplish discoloration and swelling of his toe accompanied by foul-smelling drainage. He developed gangrene. Ultimately the toe was amputated for multiple reasons. A possibly poor choice of a long day of walking had resulted in a very poor outcome.

Day after day I see diabetic patients who have walked all day in non-diabetic shoes at an amusement park or, worse yet, walked barefoot in their house or yard. Because they have no feeling in their feet, they can sustain an injury due to overuse or impalement of a tack or nail. They sometimes walk all day with a nail in their foot and do not know it! Both of these situations, in a diabetic patient, are an invitation to disaster in a diabetic patient. However, more commonly, disasters happen every day to people who did neither of these things. Over a longer period of time, let's say on the order of days to weeks, the callus, which formed from everyday wear from too much pressure on one area of the foot, can turn into an infection because the skin of a callus is not normal and is prone to invasion by bacteria. If not cared for properly, this infection ultimately can lead to an amputation. That result is every diabetic patient's worst nightmare. One amputation can lead to another amputation higher up. The wound from an amputation is as hard to heal as the initial one and I have seen it hundreds of times. If the same underlying problems exist that led to the first failure, the new wound with the same high blood sugars very well may lead to another failure.

Let's look at the processes that will help the average diabetic person protect themselves from infections.

1. The first will involve weight, diet and cholesterol control.
2. The blood sugar will need to be managed in a tight control.
3. The skin and feet will need to be monitored and cared for better than before.
4. Smoking must be off the table completely.

If all of these conditions are in place and supervised by a general physician or endocrinologist and a podiatrist, the chances for infection will be minimized.

As stated above, type 2 diabetes is often weight related. It is a well-known fact that simple weight loss will improve blood sugar control. Fat cells (especially those of diabetic patients) secrete substances that inhibit your body's ability to control blood sugar. I have had many patients who were requiring oral medications or insulin to control their blood sugar, who, with a modest amount of weight loss, they have been able to lower or stop the medications because their blood sugar came under better control. In addition, the weight that is lost is now no longer creating pressure on the feet during walking. Therefore, the first step must be weight loss for type 2 diabetic patients. If you are on medications for diabetes, be careful of low blood sugars (hypoglycemia) that may result from the better control and because of the change in diet.

I think that we have well established above that higher blood sugars are part of the problem, and that better control will improve your protection. This should be accomplished with the help from your physician. Hemoglobin A1c level is an average blood sugar over 3 months and provides a goal to reach of less than 6.0. If you are having problems getting your hemoglobin A1c below 6, or are experiencing low blood sugars, perhaps an endocrinologist would help improve the situation. With the blood sugar control and weight loss may come some improvement in high cholesterol, but, if not, the LDL cholesterol should be controlled with medications to less than 100 and most set a far lower target. Even if you can discontinue your diabetes medications because of better control of weight and diet, you are still a diabetic and you still need to monitor your feet and your cholesterol.

There are hundreds of fad diets for diabetes and weight control. Some diets can be harmful to your health. A plant based diet can lower cholesterol, promote weight loss, and reverse the effects of diabetes. This diet potentially can reverse peripheral vascular and heart disease. However, you must maintain strict willpower to keep on track as you will find that this diet is the most difficult you have ever tried. Beware the Atkins diet, as well as other popular fad diets. Carbohydrate control is only half the battle. Cholesterol levels often increase on a low carbohydrate and high fat diet. In a look at multiple studies of patients on this type of diet, all-cause mortality increased for those on the diet.

Monitoring the skin, especially that of the feet is of utmost importance. An inspection of the skin should occur every night before bedtime, looking for calluses and fungal infection. Do not ignore that callus and always wear diabetic orthotic shoes if you have peripheral neuropathy - Never walk barefoot!! Consult a podiatrist to trim the callus which will help it heal. After trimming, watch for infection because it is exceedingly common. If directed by your podiatrist, cleanse your feet daily in sterile water and dry them completely. Tinea pedis, a fungal infection of the feet (also called athlete's foot), has the appearance of scaling, dry, or peeling skin especially occurring between the toes. Use an antifungal cream at the direction of your podiatrist. These breaks in the skin (the peeling), if not treated, can allow bacteria from the surface of the skin to invade and cause a skin infection which can then invade deeper. Your nails being trimmed and free of fungal infection called onychomycosis is important also. There are prescription and over the counter medications that may help with fungal infections of the foot.

Calluses should be treated by a podiatrist. Remember, a callus is a wound waiting to happen because the skin of a callus is porous and is not protective. It is an attempt by the body to respond to excessive pressure in the area of a bony prominence, such as a toe or the ball of the foot. It consists of excess dead keratin from the layers of skin. Calluses should be debrided down to the healthier skin or to the wound that is below. Almost always there is one lurking below!! Before this is done, the podiatrist does an assessment of the blood supply by assessing the pulses or performing an ultrasound of the leg arteries to make sure the resulting wound will heal. Any time a diabetic patient has a callus or wound, unless there are good pulses, an ultrasound of the arteries should be done to assure good blood flow.

I have heard a few patients claim the podiatrist caused the wound when he shaved off some callus. What many do not understand is, as discussed above, there likely was a wound already present under the callus. After the debridement, exquisite wound care must take place to heal the opening. All of the other three processes of blood sugar, cholesterol, and weight loss must remain ideal to prevent infection. The wound care should have as its goal to increase wound healing and decrease bacterial colonization using topical silver compounds or other compounds to control bacterial growth in the surface of the wound.

Another way to prevent the increased pressure besides weight loss (but not in place of) is better footwear. Diabetic shoes possess a combination of fit, cushion and higher quality materials that help prevent calluses, foot ulcers and infections. There are other shoes that podiatrists use to off load or decrease the pressure on an area that is concerning, such as an ulcer. These are usually custom made to fit precisely. Decreasing the pressure will help the area heal faster and prevent infection.

Lastly you must quit smoking to prevent loss of toes, feet or limbs. Each puff of smoke has carbon monoxide, which will poison nerves, infection-fighting cells, and wound healing cells. Carbon monoxide also robs the distal skin of toes of vital oxygen that it needs to survive. Nicotine is the one of the culprits in the clamping down on the blood vessels mentioned above, so electronic cigarettes will not help as much as quitting altogether. E-cigarettes will, however, eliminate the carbon monoxide and low oxygen in the blood that occurs while smoking as long as the lungs are still healthy enough to function.

Lastly, peripheral arterial disease must be diagnosed early and corrected. Arterial ultrasound can detect blockages of larger arteries, which can be corrected with procedures. Often, however, diabetic patients have disease of the small arteries in the feet that cannot be remedied. This is called small vessel disease and the best you can do is control the diabetes, smoking, and cholesterol issues as tightly as possible. So even if someone tells you that your arteries are fine because the arterial ultrasound is normal, if you have diabetes, the smaller vessels are likely not normal. An arterial ultrasound only detects blockages that can be fixed by surgery or procedures. A clue to the actual degree of small vessel disease is a measurement called the ankle brachial index (ABI).

Urinary tract infections also occur frequently in diabetic patients, likely partially due to the immune system issues above. However, this cannot be the entire story. As discussed in the chapter on UTI's, the bladder muscle must completely empty the bladder to prevent infections. The peripheral neuropathy of diabetes can manifest itself as decreased bladder muscle strength and control. This then causes incomplete bladder emptying or incontinence. Diabetic patients also have urine that has excess glucose, which is the reason that, in the old days, doctors tasted the urine to diagnose diabetes. This is ripe food for the bacteria that are present in small numbers in the bladder. As with any dark, warm, and wet space with food for bacteria, the result will be infection.

As with foot infections, part of your protection will be blood sugar control, but improving the urinary bladder emptying will also be important. Weight loss may improve emptying, but the most important step may be seeing an urologist, who would perform emptying and flow studies to help find the cause of the bladder function issues. There are treatments for prostate obstruction problems and for nerve damage. Consulting with an urologist is useful anytime you have frequent urinary tract infections as a diabetic.

Pneumonia, bloodstream infections, and a host of other infections also occur more frequently in diabetic patients and these infections are discussed elsewhere in this book. In summary, the path to protecting yourself from infections in diabetes will always be blood sugar, weight, and cholesterol control. In addition, smoking cessation and exquisite foot care are essential to save your toes and limbs from the surgeon's block.

More information:

http://www.prevention.com/health/diabetes/preventions-5-week-diabetes-diet-meal-plan

http://www.forksoverknives.com

http://www.niddk.nih.gov/health-information/diabetes/preventing-diabetes-problems/keep-feet-healthy

http://www.diabetes.org/living-with-diabetes/complications/

Chapter 8

~

Clostridium difficile Infections

It was her third episode in 6 months of this diarrheal illness that was so horrific that she did not leave her bathroom for 3 days. What began as a simple antibiotic given for a cough resulted in a *Clostridium difficile* infection, or what is commonly called C diff, an illness that caused 30 pounds of weight loss on an already small elderly frame. Luckily for her a new procedure to add the bacteria from the intestines of a group of donors had been available at this hospital and after a few days of antibiotics to treat her infection, she was given a fecal microbiota transplant. A 6 month ordeal had finally ended and she would go on to put on some weight and was getting around better within a few weeks.

This epidemic has been killing thousands of people per year and it is rarely talked about, though many of my elderly patients have heard of someone who has contracted it. Since approximately the years 2000 to 2001, two resistant and more virulent strains of an intestinal bacteria spread first from the US, then from Canada, around the world. Much more deadly than the previously known strain of a bacterium known as *Clostridium difficile*, these strains produced more toxin and were particularly deadly for the elderly. What is remarkable is that this bacterium probably evolved and rapidly spread because of our overuse of a class of antibiotic called fluoroquinolones and our lack of an effective infection control strategy for this bacteria. It rapidly spread because it could be harbored in the intestines of healthy persons without symptoms.

How was such a deadly bacteria able to hide but spread so effectively? The bacteria in your intestines act like multiple bullies on a playground, in that these bacteria are constantly at war with each other. The constant battles and the energy that they expend in this warfare prevent any one of them from becoming very powerful. If you remove one bully's enemies, this will upset the applecart, and the enemy bully will become too powerful. There are a billion bacteria in your intestines and there are more than 1000 species of bacteria. The vast majority of these bacteria are good bacteria that do not harm the host, but instead provide us with assistance in digesting our foods and maintaining the health of our intestines. Even for most harmful bacteria, it usually takes a large amount of the bacteria to be ingested to cause illness, or it requires the good bacteria to be knocked down so that the harmful bacteria can proliferate more easily.

Antibiotics and other factors can alter the types of bacteria found in our intestines. You see, antibiotics don't just kill the bacteria they are intended to kill, they destroy millions of bacteria in the intestines after you swallow them and prior to their absorption into your system. Only about 40 to 95% of the ingested antibiotics get absorbed, leaving the rest to travel the length of your intestines, killing innocent by-standing bacteria. As a result, there is an over-abundance of the remaining bacteria which could cause symptoms, such as diarrhea. This is one of the reasons that antibiotics commonly cause diarrhea.

Clostridium difficile is one such bacterium that is normally found in the intestines of about 6 to 10% of a normal population. It has been found in the intestines of persons of every age, from neonates to the elderly without causing any symptoms. It has become resistant to several antibiotics including the most commonly prescribed group of antibiotics called fluoroquinolones. Therefore when you take certain antibiotics, they will not kill the C diff in your intestines. If the C diff survives, and the other bacteria are killed by the antibiotic, then the C diff will be free to grow unchecked. It will then coat the inside of the colon, causing inflammation and may potentially cause a severe and sometimes fatal infection.

Other risk factors for C diff disease are age, female sex, and a weakened immune system. Age is such a strong risk factor that 1 in 1000 persons over 65 will contract C diff each year, while 1 in 100 persons over 85 will suffer from the illness each year. Death occurs from C diff more likely if the patient is older or if there is a weakened immune system. The risk of death is up to 35%, depending on the severity of the illness.

In addition to antibiotics, proton pump inhibitors (PPI) such as omeprazole, esomeprazole, pantoprazole, and lansoprazole can increase the risk of *Clostridium difficile* infection. These medications decrease the acid in your stomach to the degree that the *Clostridium difficile* bacteria, when ingested, will be more likely to survive the passage through the acidic stomach to reach the large intestines which is where they cause their damage. There are millions of patients that do not need to be on PPI and could be on H2 inhibitors like ranitidine or famotidine for treatment of their gastroesophageal reflux disease (GERD). H2 inhibitors may not decrease the acid to the point of negating the protective effect of the acid in your stomach, but enough for reduction of symptoms of most people. PPIs were not meant for long-term usage and there are multiple possible side effects and adverse events associated with long-term use. However, for peptic or duodenal ulcers and significant reflux not responding to other therapies, they are absolutely necessary.

Nasogastric tubes are tubes that are inserted through the nose that pass through the stomach into the small intestines. Similar to the risk of PPIs, if bacteria are ingested through the tube, they can bypass the acid of the stomach and are more likely to survive the passage. If the end of the tube that the liquid feeding tube connection is not clean or has been contaminated by the hands of healthcare workers, C diff can easily gain entry to the intestines.

During my training from 1998 to 2003, C diff was an uncommon infection at the busy hospitals in which I was learning. After training, as a director of infection control, I have seen C diff increase in numbers from 100,000 hospitalizations per year around the year 2000 to more than 300,000 hospitalizations in 2010. Overall there are approximately 700,000 C diff infections per year in the US. In addition, the severity has increased because the strain that causes almost half of the illnesses is a stronger more virulent strain. It pumps out 1000 times more toxin into the intestines than the other strains, causing much more inflammation and thus more severe disease. The fatality of the disease has increased from a total of 800 deaths in 1999 to about 8,000 in 2008. In the elderly the fatality rate is very high, as more than 93% of the deaths in 2008 occurred in those over 65. A person who is over 85 has a 35% likelihood of dying if they contract the disease.

Clostridium difficile colonizes the intestines in two forms. The first is the active form or vegetative form. The second is the dormant spore form. The active form can stay alive on moist surfaces for several hours and is killed by stomach acid. It forms toxins that create the disease in humans called pseudomembranous colitis, mentioned above. The spore form can remain in the intestines for weeks, is not killed by antibiotics and can remain viable on dry surfaces for weeks. Swallowing this form in sufficient quantities, due to its ability to survive the acidic environment of the stomach, will create colonization. As mentioned before, colonization is normal and 6 to 10 percent of the population has this bacteria living in their intestines among the billions of other bacteria.

Once colonized the patient can then develop disease if that bacteria can overtake the rest of the bacteria in the intestines and coat the inside of the colon. It can do this if there is sufficient disruption of the normal bacteria, such as with antibiotic usage or another diarrheal illness. Diminished immune function with age may also be contributing to its ability to cause disease. Once the *C. difficile* dominates the flora it forms yellow gray membranes (think of this as a layer of slime) on the walls of the intestines. There is marked inflammation in the colon, which causes abdominal pain, nausea and mucus-laden stool (often yellow with a peculiar odor recognized by healthcare workers) with frequent crampy diarrhea.

The infection control nightmare at hospitals and in homes owes to the hardiness of the spores of C diff. C diff is not killed by alcohol gel or foams or most soaps. However, washing hands with soap and water is the most effective means for healthcare workers or caregivers to prevent the spread to others. The going theory is that the water physically rinses the spores from the hands down the drain. C diff is killed on surfaces by using a dilute bleach solution (1 cup bleach in 2 gallons of water). Make sure you rinse the area after it stands for at least 10 minutes and only use in a well-ventilated area. Similar compounds are used to clean the rooms and equipment of C diff patients after use in hospitals.

It has been well established that a person is more likely to contract the illness caused by *Clostridium difficile* if he or she receives antibiotics. A recent study showed that if a patient, who occupied the bed just prior to a second patient, received antibiotics, the second patient was more likely to contract C diff infection. Along with a myriad of other evidence, this would suggest that, the *Clostridium difficile* is either already in your intestines, or it is acquired while you are in the hospital from the environment in your room.

The issue with C diff infection at home, is that it is likely all over the house of an infected patient. It may also be in the bathrooms of colonized (presence of the bacteria without symptoms) patients. From the bathroom to the kitchen, with frequent bowel movements and presence on the skin, this bacteria and its spores will be everywhere. In the bedroom, the bacterium can be found on sheets and even on clean clothes. In the bathroom especially, spores will be on toilets, floors, sinks, towels, and showers. This presents a high likelihood of colonization of family members. It is highly recommended that these areas be cleaned with a dilute bleach solution to prevent either family members or the patient themselves from acquiring or reacquiring the bacteria.

Probiotics continue to increase in popularity, likely owing to the homeopathic movement in the world and the widespread commercials featuring celebrities espousing the benefits of these over the counter products. It keeps them "regular" they say, but the benefits go far beyond that. The bacteria that are in probiotics vary from *Bifidobacterium* to *Lactobacillus*. These are the same bacteria that are present in most commercially developed yogurts. There is a yeast that is used in one product also, *Saccharomyces boulardii*. While not proven to prevent *Clostridium difficile* infection, probiotics have been proven to prevent the diarrhea associated with antibiotics not caused by C difficile. It is logical to assume that there must be some modest benefit to taking probiotics in preventing C difficile.

So what can you do to protect yourself from *Clostridium difficile* infections? Decrease usage of antibiotics and PPIs as directed by your physician. If you have to take either class of medication, then take probiotics to replenish your gut bacteria if recommended by your physician. Again, there is a small risk of complications in certain patients taking probiotics consult your physician.

Given that half of all C diff infections occur in nursing facilities and hospitals, special attention to your space in these locations is important. See the chapters on hospitals and nursing facilities for more information, but if you are hospitalized or are having surgery, wash your hands often and use bleach wipes to clean your personal space when you first get there and every day if you are allowed. This includes the bedrails, tray table, bathroom, chairs, and the nurse call/TV remote. It is important to clean this way to prevent accidental ingestion of the bacteria. New sheets should be used every day. The floors and bathroom should be cleaned by housekeeping every day. Ask your nurses or doctor questions about antibiotic and PPI use. Are they necessary? If you require a nasogastric tube (a tube in the stomach through the nose), and are receiving feeding through the tube, be aware of what goes in the tube and keep the end clean.

If you or a loved one has C diff, use a bleach cleaner to clean the house and use bleach and hot water to clean the sheets and the individual's clothes. Use gloves when handling linens or when cleaning. Use soap and water to wash your hands before and after cleaning. If your immune system is suppressed, ask your doctor about any other protections that might be available.

For more information:

Lessa FC, Gould CV, McDonald LC. Current Status of Clostridium difficile Infection Epidemiology. Clinical Infectious Diseases: An Official Publication of the Infectious Diseases Society of America. 2012;55(Suppl 2):S65-S70. doi:10.1093/cid/cis319. **http://www.ncbi.nlm.nih.gov/ pubmed/22752867**

Freeman J, et al. The Changing Epidemiology of Clostridium Difficile Infections. Clin. Microbiol. Rev. July 2010 vol. 23 no. 3 529-549. **http:// cmr.asm.org/content/23/3/529.full**

http://www.cdc.gov/HAI/organisms/cdiff/Cdiff_infect.html

http://cid.oxfordjournals.org/content/50/12/e77.full

Chapter 9

~

Diverticulitis

Everyone above age 50 should read this chapter, because it is very likely you have this condition called diverticulosis and do not know it. Diverticulosis is an out pouching of the large intestine like a weak wall of an old bicycle tire inner tube. That wall will form a balloon like a bubble on the edge of the tire tube. If this happens in the colon, then that bubble will have feces within it, and consequently millions of bacteria. Diverticulosis is not such a problem, other than that these pouches do not carry feces quickly out of the body and could create an area of bacterial overgrowth. The condition of diverticulosis is very common as we get older because the muscles that run lengthwise and circumferentially around the colon become weaker. That weak area with no muscular layer could allow an out pouching described above. A healthy colon keeps feces and bacteria moving toward the exit. Any stagnant areas will cause bacterial overgrowth and this can create abdominal symptoms ranging from flatulence to bloating and pain.

If that pocket that lies outside the intestinal tube becomes pinched off from the rest of the colon and cannot readily drain back into the colon, then the bacteria inside the pocket will grow unchecked causing an infection called diverticulitis. The symptoms of this illness are left lower abdominal pain, nausea, fever, and intermittent diarrhea and constipation. The pain is usually localized to the lower left because the left side of the colon is more likely to have the out pouchings called diverticuli. If the bacteria grow enough, they can burst or perforate the pocket and gain access to the area outside the colon called the peritoneum. This forms an abscess or peritonitis and an even more severe infection called sepsis. Diverticulitis can often be treated as an outpatient but once it becomes an abscess it may need to be treated in the hospital with intravenous antibiotics.

The goal for prevention of diverticulitis is to keep the flow of fecal matter moving toward the exit. Think of the crowd trying to exit the theater. The people in the back are pushing the people in front out the door. If 20 of these people suddenly are diverted into a broom closet, it won't be long before they find their way out if the door remains open. But if the door to the closet closes, those 20 people will not be happy and will get quite agitated. After a few hours the odors and sweating will be unbearable. They will be climbing out the windows if given a chance. If you can keep the people moving toward the exit, they will be less likely to be diverted into the closet.

Keeping the stool flowing will keep the diverticulum open and bacteria that flow in will also flow out. In addition, constipation causes straining with bowel movements, which increases pressure inside the colon, similar to the way increased pressure inside the bicycle tire tube will increase the size of the bubble. Rate of flow (constipation or diarrhea) is affected by different factors such as diet, hydration, types of bacteria present, obesity, age, and medications. A diet higher in fiber tends to lead to less constipation and more stool flow. Dehydration leads the body to reabsorb more water from the intestines causing more constipation. It is obvious that eliminating constipation is necessary for flow, but sometimes it is a difficult task to avoid constipation. Taking stool softeners and consuming a high fiber diet will help with the flow and ease of the colon pushing the stool forward. Though controversial, there is a concept that ingesting small, hard particle foods such as popcorn and nuts and seeds (or fruits with seeds such as strawberries) increases the chance of obstructing the entrance and exit of the diverticulum.

I can tell you that, anecdotally, I have heard from many patients that they ate popcorn just several hours before their symptoms began. One of them was a friend who had popcorn about 18 hours before her left lower abdominal pain and took a few days of antibiotics before the pain subsided. I have encountered many patients in the hospital with severe abdominal pain and fever. About 5 percent of these patients require surgery such as another gentleman that I saw recently who had a perforated abscess and this was not getting better with antibiotics. The abscess kept getting larger on each of the CT scans that we did a few days apart from each other. This patient required surgery to remove that part of the colon surrounding the diverticulum. At the same time, in the same hospital, was a female who had three previous episodes of diverticulitis in the previous year that improved with antibiotics by mouth. She was started on intravenous antibiotics after admitting to the hospital and, due to the recurrences, also underwent a similar procedure. Some of the patients who undergo this procedure have a colostomy placed, which means for a few months they have a plastic pouch on the outside of their abdomen that receives and collects stool. So you can see that prevention can be very important to prevent these complicated scenarios involving surgery.

Protecting yourself will involve a change in your diet and habits that will not be easy. The easiest change may be the use of probiotics. Probiotics may help prevent diverticulitis by increasing the beneficial digestion of materials in the intestines and consequently diminishing constipation. Conversely, there are diets, medications, and other toxins that may disrupt the normal bacteria populations (flora) in the intestines and may promote diverticulitis to a small degree. Older persons are more likely to have diverticulosis and are more likely to have constipation. They are also more likely to have disrupted bacterial flora either due to poor diet, obesity or frequent antibiotic use. Obesity increases the straining that must occur for a bowel movement due to the lack of an effective stomach wall musculature. Both older and obese patients also tend to eat less fiber.

Medications can also promote diverticulitis. Pain and anxiety medications, calcium and iron supplements, antihistamines, calcium channel blocking blood pressure medications, and other medications can increase constipation. Antibiotics, chemotherapy, and immune suppressant medications may alter the bacterial flora, thus promoting diverticulitis. Some diuretic medications such as furosemide and hydrochlorothiazide may trend the body toward dehydration and cause constipation. Alcohol can cause constipation by both dehydration and decreased strength of colon muscle contractions.

The evidence for using a high fiber diet is plentiful. In some non-European societies that have high fiber diets, diverticulosis is far less common than in countries such as England and the US, where we eat a lower fiber diet. In countries in Southeast Asia, there is a very low incidence of diverticulitis owing to high fiber, low fat, and relatively meatless diets. Those with diet higher in fiber have lower stool transit times, i.e. it takes less time for food to exit the intestines and therefore there is less time to reabsorb water, and therefore the stool is softer.

The path to protecting yourself from diverticulitis involves increased fiber and water in the diet and decreasing constipation. Your diet should contain at least 35 grams of fiber per day. Probiotics may also be taken. Avoiding ingestion of seeds and nuts is controversial and there is no scientific evidence to support the recommendation. However, there are a lot of anecdotal reports of patients eating certain foods and having an attack of diverticulitis. The problem is that these foods may be part of a high fiber diet that is recommended and one study (a cohort study and not a blinded one which limits its usefulness) suggests that persons who ate nuts and seeds were less likely to have diverticulosis diagnosed and less likely to come down with an attack of diverticulitis. At this point, in general the recommendation would be if you have had occurrences associated with certain foods, then avoid those foods. If so, foods to potentially avoid include (but are not limited to) strawberries, blueberries, raspberries, blackberries, popcorn, nuts, tomatoes, and coconut.

Other recommendations are geared toward increasing the flow and minimizing constipation. Staying well hydrated with water is an important part of this. Your mother's nagging recommendation for 6 glasses of water per day is actually true in this regard. Pain medications increase constipation, and if you are on these medications, you should ask your physician how to prevent constipation. Limiting sugar intake and decreasing weight can also help in this endeavor.

With better flow and higher fiber diet, the risk of diverticulitis will be minimized. Medications could be changed if constipation is still present despite a high fiber diet. Alcohol intake should also be minimized. There are multiple studies suggesting exercise is associated with a decreased risk of developing both diverticulosis and diverticulitis. A light exercise program may also help with constipation also and is easy to initiate, but difficult to maintain. If you are overweight, weight loss is also recommended. Hopefully these measures will help prevent further issues in your health.

More Information:

http://www.ucsfhealth.org/education/diverticular_disease_and_diet/

Chapter 10

❧

Influenza and Pneumonia

She was one of the many in 2009 who had contracted H1N1 influenza. She was young, only 29 years old and already an accomplished teacher. That was the hallmark of this outbreak, that those who were worst affected were the young and not older people. She came in to the hospital only 24 hours after the onset of the symptoms of fever, chills and shortness of breath. She was already on a breathing machine and was clinically worsening with a positive test for influenza. She was immediately started on antibiotics and an antiviral for influenza. It took 2 weeks in the hospital and about a month in a rehabilitation center to recover, and it was 6 months before she felt anywhere close to back to normal. This situation continues to happen though less frequently than 2009, where a severe form of influenza attacks otherwise healthy individuals.

Unlike the rest of the world where malaria and tuberculosis are the biggest infectious disease killers, in the United States, between 5 and 10% of all deaths are caused by the combination of influenza and pneumonia. The two are lumped together because influenza often is not diagnosed but presumed to be the cause of a portion of pneumonia illnesses. Influenza and other viral infections, such as adenovirus, can also be the culprit of pneumonia (viral and post-viral pneumonia) and may be the most common cause of pneumonia. It is said that pneumonia is the friend of the old man, but having seen many deaths from pneumonia it is not the friend that it would seem. Robbing the body of oxygen, the shortness of breath and chest pain accompanying the pneumonia is not a comfortable way to die.

Pneumonia can be caused by several viruses or bacteria. Among the viruses causing pneumonia are influenza, adenovirus, parainfluenza, respiratory syncytial virus, and metapneumovirus. The most common bacterial cause is *Streptococcus pneumoniae* also called pneumococcus. Other bacteria include *Haemophilus influenzae, Klebsiella pneumoniae*, and *Staphylococcus*. A subset of pneumonia called "atypical pneumonia" can be caused by *Legionella, Mycoplasma pneumoniae* or *Chlamydophila pneumoniae* among others. Some of these bacteria and viruses are contagious and some are acquired from the environment.

Aspiration pneumonia occurs when bacteria from the mouth or throat are accidentally allowed into the lungs. This can occur during a vomiting episode or while a person is unconscious, inebriated, or in a much weakened state. Aspiration pneumonia is extremely common in the elderly and occurs most frequently in nursing facilities and hospitals where people are at their weakest with a different illness. Post-obstructive pneumonia occurs when cancer obstructs part of an airway, causing the lung's inability to clear secretions and bacteria from the other side of the obstruction.

I frequently hear, "How did I get pneumonia if I had the pneumonia shot?" As you can see from the previous few paragraphs, which is nowhere near complete, there are more causes of pneumonia than just *Streptococcus pneumoniae*, which is the only bacterium covered by the pneumonia shot. And it only protects you from 13 or 23 strains of pneumococcal pneumonia depending on the brand name of the vaccine.

Risk factors for pneumonia include advanced age, emphysema, smoking, neurologic disorders, poor nutrition status, malignancy, and recent surgery. As mentioned before, a viral infection can lead to bacterial pneumonia, hence the term post-viral pneumonia. Classically this is a two phase illness where viral symptoms present first, followed by a period of the patient feeling better, and ultimately followed by worsening fever, productive cough, and shortness of breath. This is probably more common than we think because often the two phases are indistinguishable. Sometimes there is a gradual worsening in post-viral pneumonia. Therefore, if we want to protect ourselves from pneumonia, we need to be thinking viruses, including the common cold viruses and influenza.

Influenza virus is a very common virus that often leads to pneumonia and is very preventable. We can learn from the history of epidemics to see how devastating it can be. Every 1-3 years we have an epidemic of a novel influenza strain that spreads rapidly and every 20 years we have a pandemic that affects a majority of the population. The most cited epidemic, because it was so deadly, is the Influenza Epidemic of 1918. It started in a military base in Kansas, and within 9 months 600,000 Americans died and there were 20 million deaths worldwide. Influenza killed more people during World War I than warfare. There were casket shortages and mass funerals. The most recent illnesses with H1N1 Influenza starting in 2009 has also had a big impact on the population, and we are continuing to see these infections many years later.

A good portion of the rest of pneumonia is caused by aspiration. Arguably, all pneumonia is due to aspiration, since the bacteria must migrate from the back of the throat to the airways in some manner. Normally there are bacteria that exist in the upper airways of the lung, but the ciliary (small hairs on cells which brush outward) motion of the cells lining the airways sweeps the bacteria out of the lungs. In patients with emphysema, smoking, and conditions causing weakness, this ciliary motion is impaired or lacking. Nicotine and toxins and carbon monoxide poison the ciliary cells. Frank aspiration occurs when weakness of the muscles which keep the epiglottis closed over the opening of the trachea causes enough saliva or stomach secretions to enter into the lungs overcoming the ciliary action.

The strength and nutrition of the elderly is of utmost importance. Certainly obesity increases the risk of pneumonia, but being underweight can also affect your ability to survive pneumonia. It is extremely common for the elderly to become thin and malnourished. If this is happening to you or a loved one, you must do everything in your power to prevent the slow downward spiral by increasing nutrition and strength. One convincing statistic to use is the Body Mass Index (BMI). Elderly patients with a BMI below 23 have 1.8 times the risk of developing infections including pneumonia. There are online websites available to calculate your BMI. It is important to have significant protein and fat in the diet as well as a calcium and Vitamin D supplement. The diet should have at least 2400 calories per day if someone is below a BMI of 18. Nutritional drinks often help with the calories and nutrients.

Maintaining strength and fitness is crucial including both lower and upper body strength. Too many people think that the walking they do during the day is sufficient. Some cardiovascular exercise such as brisk walking is more effective. Water aerobics is a popular activity for older persons and usually includes upper body strength with water weights if you are strong enough. If the person is in a hospital or nursing facility, spending as much time out of bed in a chair or walking is extremely important. Even sitting in a chair increases the use of muscles that will help prevent pneumonia. The use of wheelchairs or motorized scooters, while they help with the ability of persons to get around, may not be doing them any favors with respect to strength. Avoiding the use of a scooter, if approved by a physician, should be undertaken. These scooters are often used due to orthopedic reasons so sometimes they are not avoidable.

Now, let's talk about how to further protect yourself from pneumonia. We said before that to protect yourself you must prevent viral infections and aspiration. Frequent hand washing or hand sanitizing with alcohol gel is important to keep viral infections in check, especially in the elderly. This is extremely important around children who can spread viruses even when they are not sick. Children are commonly the ones spreading viral illnesses (even when they are not sick) so taking the utmost care in avoiding the germs associated with them is difficult but a necessity. Vaccinating children for influenza is an important way to prevent pneumonia in older adults. If you have a family member stricken with a viral infection you should wash your hands frequently and wear a mask. The affected family member should wash their hands frequently as well.

Preventing aspiration pneumonia involves consulting a speech therapist if you have had a stroke or if there is such profound weakness that you are bed bound. The speech therapist can perform tests to determine if there is a swallowing problem. They will teach some methods to protect you from aspirating. First, never tilt your head back while swallowing as this keeps the epiglottis open, allowing food or saliva to enter the lungs. Instead, tilt the chin down toward the chest when swallowing. Using straws is a danger because in order to suck on the straw you need to keep the epiglottis open, and if the liquid is drawn in too quickly it will also go down the windpipe. If using a straw is necessary, separate the technique into two stages. First suck the liquid into the mouth, taking care to not allow any liquid past the tongue. Then, remove the straw from the mouth and, while performing the chin tilt maneuver, begin to move the liquid down the throat. Taking smaller bites and taking time to chew adequately also will help. Another situation I see every day - the weak patient is lying in bed, half-reclined, eating a meal in the hospital. Never allow this to happen to a loved one. They need to be sitting up straight to avoid inhaling their food and drink. If there is a swallowing disorder, the speech therapist may recommend using a thickener for thin liquids because thickened liquids are less likely to go directly down the airway.

Vaccinations are the most important protection against influenza and pneumonia. If you have the influenza vaccine annually you decrease your risk of acquiring the flu by up to 60%. If you are over 65, influenza vaccination reduces your chances of being hospitalized for pneumonia by 20% and overall mortality is reduced by 30-60%. The influenza vaccination should be taken in September to October before the flu season starts. At the present time there are two influenza vaccines with either 3 or 4 vaccine components called trivalent or quadrivalent. For those concerned about mercury and thimerosal, there are preservative-free options. There is also a higher strength formulation for older adults. They are all effective, but ask your doctor which one is best for you.

Let's go over the reasons people avoid influenza vaccinations. The biggest reason I hear is that the individual says, "I got the flu" or "I got sick" after getting vaccinated. Fever and myalgia (muscle aches) are common after vaccinations and these are not unlike flu symptoms. The illness is almost always mild and is better than having the actual flu. My reply for this discussion is that you can protect yourself, your children, your parents, and your friends from a potentially deadly illness. If you are younger, you are less likely to die, but it may not be just you that you should be thinking about. People can carry influenza and not know that they are spreading it, and if you are around an elderly person, you can spread the infection to them. Therefore, the real protection of your flu vaccination is gained by your older friends and relatives.

Many people completely underestimate the impact that influenza has on the population. They think that they never get the flu, so why should they get the vaccine? I used to hear this from nurses who wanted to avoid the vaccine in the hospital. However, a well-timed lecture showing the casket shortages of 1918, and showing the effect on their patients, usually increased the rate of healthcare workers receiving the vaccine. Even better now, is requiring healthcare workers to receive the vaccine or they have to wear a mask the entire flu season.

There are two pneumonia vaccinations, each with their own strengths, one that protects you from 23 strains of pneumococcus (the most common cause of pneumonia) and one that protects from 13 strains. The 13 strain vaccine has a better (or at least different) method of strengthening your immune system against the bacteria. The official recommendations regarding these 2 vaccinations for pneumonia are still evolving, but at this point, it is recommended to have both vaccinations at least once after age 65 a year apart. If you have certain illnesses including diabetes or heart disease you should receive these vaccines earlier – this is important to discuss with your physician!

One final vaccine that is important is the Tdap vaccine which protects you from tetanus, diphtheria, and pertussis. Pertussis is becoming so important in the elderly as the memory of their immune system forgets about the previous vaccination they had in young adulthood. Pertussis in the elderly can lead to pneumonia and may be involved in a small but important portion of overall pneumonia because the complications in the elderly are increased. See the chapter on pertussis for more information.

In summary, to protect yourself from pneumonia involves nutrition and strength if you are elderly and always includes both the influenza and the pneumonia vaccines. If you are hospitalized, keeping up strength and nutrition are major goals of your recovery. Always keep your head of your bed elevated if you are at risk for aspiration. Outside of the hospital, be aware of those who have illnesses around you and avoid them. Have all of your loved ones from the youngest children to the elderly vaccinated against influenza. Frequent hand washing is important as it could prevent the spread of the bacteria and viruses that could make you ill.

For More Information:

http://www.cdc.gov/flu/about/qa/publications.htm

http://www.cdc.gov/flu/about/disease/65over.htm

https://www.cdc.gov/vaccines/vpd-vac/pneumo/

Chapter 11

~

Sexually Transmitted Diseases and HIV

Sexually transmitted diseases (STDs) have been around since the days of the caveman and they remain today as hidden and taboo in everyday discussions despite their widespread prevalence. They may not admit it publicly, but close to 50% of persons above age 18 in the United States have had an STD. The reasons we do not protect ourselves from these maladies are as unknown as the reasons we do not protect ourselves from many illnesses. It is this sense of invincibility that makes us think we will not contract cancer when we smoke, have liver disease if we drink, and contract venereal diseases if we have unprotected sex.

According to blood tests, approximately 15-20% of the US population has been exposed and therefore continue to shed Herpes simplex virus type 2 (genital herpes). In 2012, according to the CDC, there were 1,400,000 cases of chlamydia, 334,000 cases of gonorrhea, and 45,000 cases of syphilis diagnosed in the US. Human Papillomavirus (HPV), which causes genital warts and is implicated in penis, cervix, anal and oral cancers, has been found in 23% of all individuals, and 35% of younger women age 14-19. To round out the STDs, there were 47,000 new cases of HIV diagnosed in 2012 which brings the total of persons living with HIV or AIDS to 1.2 million in the US. According to the World Health Organization (WHO), there are 35 million persons living with HIV in the world of which 3.2 million are children. There are a few other less common noted STDs including granuloma inguinale (Donovanosis), chancroid, lymphogranuloma venereum (LGV) and a few other viruses. Trichomonas is extremely common and can be sexually transmitted but can sometimes be transmitted by non-sexual means.

90

Of particular concern in Florida and other retirement hotbeds, as the sexually liberated baby boomers retire, there is an alarming increase in STDs in the elderly. There are retirement areas of Florida with STD rates that rival the rates in those aged 15 to 20. Think about it. Sixty year old Charles or Mabel has lost his or her spouse of 40 years and suddenly finds that he or she is on the dating scene again but this time with no worries about pregnancy. With the advent of medications for erectile dysfunction, there are fewer barriers to sex after 60 than ever. Herpes, gonorrhea, chlamydia, and syphilis rates are increasing among this age group.

I always take a step back for a second when I have an elderly couple in my office and one of them asks, "Well, when did I get this herpes infection and how did my husband/wife give this to me." First I have to explain to them that the blood test that they had does not tell when the person acquired the infection. Then I have to tell them that they may have acquired it early in life with sexual intimacy, so it was not necessarily their husband of 50 years that gave it to them. There is usually a sigh of relief at this moment and then we can all relax and talk about how to manage possible outbreaks and transmission.

Statistics, though, have never been very effective at prevention for STDs. Education is helpful, but can only go so far. If you are over 30, chances are you already have an STD. The key will be to protect yourself from other STDs and to protect the next generation, educate your children early. If you ask your doctor to run an antibody blood test for herpes and HPV, there is a 40% likelihood you will turn up positive. And the person with whom you are about to have sex also has the same 40% likelihood. There is a 60% likelihood one of the two of you have an STD. The key to prevention is the understanding if you contract one or more of the number of sexually acquired infections they could actually decrease your ability to have children, you could spread it to someone else, or sometimes bring your life to an unfortunate premature end.

I have seen many destructive sexual behaviors that defy logic. I have seen people risk their lives for just the tender touch of another or the inclusion in a social group. People have actually contracted HIV on purpose just so they can be included in a group they wanted to belong. They call it gifting and receiving. One person who has HIV willingly transmits the virus to another willing recipient. Sounds impossible but true! Prostitution, online chat rooms, and cell phone dating applications that facilitate casual sex occurrence more often by promoting risky behaviors that have resulted in higher STD rates.

The younger a patient is, the less likely they are to heed any logic about STDs. I have many a patient that seems like they would rather die a thousand deaths than think about STDs and HIV. Unfortunately the hyperbole may be very accurate. The risk they are taking, to them, seems to be very small, compared to the feelings of inclusion and closeness that a sexual relationship brings them. Even with a fleeting short-term one-night stand they don't seem to grasp the risk. Including alcohol and drug use with unprotected sex causes the risk of STD infection to soar. Prevention needs to be brought more into the foreground of the minds of these individuals

At the risk of this becoming a lecture in a middle school health class, the answer to the prevention question is not any different from the answer given 20 years ago. To protect yourself from STDs you will need to prevent the transfer of the germ from one person to another; with persons having genital secretions that are possibly infected, then this means preventing the transfer of genital secretions from one person to another. Two syllables, rubber, the old term, condom – the preferred modern term. Latex is still used in condoms, so you should get acquainted or reacquainted with the device. Apart from abstinence, it is the most effective method to prevent STDs including HIV infection. Learn to carry condoms and make sure you always have a supply on hand. Douching to prevent infection, the old wives' tale, does not prevent STDs and can facilitate certain infections if done after sex.

Recognition is the next important concept. Recognition of symptoms of an STD will prevent spread to another person. Any unusual discharge or "drip" should be followed by a trip to the doctor. Women should get pelvic examinations and pap smears regularly at all ages even if they have had a hysterectomy. Pelvic examinations can diagnose gonorrhea, chlamydia, trichomonas, bacterial vaginosis and yeast infections with better accuracy now. Because these infections often do not have symptoms, the only way to diagnose them is to have regular testing. In addition, human papilloma virus can be detected during the exam now with better accuracy. Even men can and should have regular testing (as often as yearly) with a simple urine test for gonorrhea and chlamydia, along with blood tests for HIV and syphilis if they are sexually active. Men no longer have to have the fear of a medical object being stuck up into the penis to screen for STDs.

A doctor should also check out lesions on the genitals. Because syphilis and herpes are often underdiagnosed, simple blood tests should be performed every few years if you are sexually active and have any kind of lesion. If you have a genital sore but are negative for syphilis and herpes, then the ulcer can be tested for chancroid and granuloma inguinale which are rare in the US but more common elsewhere around the world, including the Caribbean close-by. If you are positive for herpes, you can take safe medications, such as the prescription medication valacyclovir, that can help prevent transmission to your sexual partner.

If you or your partner are diagnosed with an STD, abstain from sex with anyone until both of you are completely finished with your treatment regimen. For syphilis, you must abstain from sex for longer than the duration of the treatment, until your lab tests show that you have cleared the bacteria. Because syphilis can recur even after treatment, your doctor should order follow-up blood tests to make sure that the bacteria has not reappeared. If you feel uncomfortable with your primary care provider, your local health department has free or low cost STD testing. Also, Planned Parenthood has STD testing available. If you are sexually active, you should be tested at least yearly for gonorrhea, chlamydia, and HPV. If you have been diagnosed with an STD you should be tested more often.

What about the future? We can prevent the strains of HPV that cause most of the HPV related cancers with a vaccine if it is given early enough in life prior to significant sexual exposure. Make sure your sons and daughters and grandchildren get the vaccine (usually around age 11-12). HPV related cancers include cervical cancer, anal cancer and oral (tongue, mouth, and throat) cancers. Cervical cancers are decreasing because of the advent of Pap smear screening during recommended pelvic exams for women. Anal and oral cancers are increasing so rapidly they are rising in the incidence rankings. We are slowly starting to increase our awareness of oral and anal cancers and early diagnosis strategies. Hopefully with better, early diagnosis of precancerous conditions, similar to the way diagnosis of cervical dysplasia impacts cervical cancer survival, we can impact the numbers of oral and anal cancers. It is believed that in 20 years, the incidence of cervical, anal, and oral cancers will decrease because of awareness and the vaccine.

HIV used to be considered by some a disease of only gay men; however, this could not be further from the truth. Half of all new infections with the virus that causes AIDS are transmitted heterosexually. This is often diagnosed in middle-aged women, especially African-American women. The reason this virus continues to proliferate is that half of all persons who are infected with this virus do not know they have it and therefore many of these individuals continue to spread it to others. If only we could have everyone in the world tested and then get those diagnosed treated, we may be able to eradicate this virus from the earth.

Know your risk and if you do not know the status of your partner for all sexually transmitted diseases including HIV, then use a condom. Do not be afraid to ask the STD/HIV status of your partner. If you are going to be sexually active, then you both can get tested at the same time prior to sex. Testing takes less than 20 minutes and results return within that same 20 minutes. Wait for sex until this is done. You can do it. It is not worth the possible complications and possible death from an illness you could have prevented. Protect yourself first...

If you do have unprotected intercourse with someone who you think may be infected, there are ways you can prevent HIV. As we discussed above, anyone who is sexually active is at risk for being infected with HIV. There is something called post-exposure prophylaxis (PEP) which if started within 24 to 48 hours after sex may prevent HIV infection. The chances of preventing HIV are better if you take the medication sooner after exposure and you take all doses as prescribed. There is also pre-exposure prophylaxis (PrEP) for persons who engage in high risk behavior or are a partner of someone with HIV. Taking a single pill daily could prevent HIV infection. PrEP is not 100% effective, so condom use is still required, and even then there is no guarantee you could not become infected. The chances of prevention with PrEP is also tied to compliance with the drug regimen with no missed doses. Neither of these protects you 100% from all other STD's. You will need to ask your doctor about these possibilities.

Whatever you do, just being more aware of the risks out there makes you more informed and better able to be your own protector. Remembering that you are more valuable than the love you seek will help keep you out of trouble.

For more information:

http://www.cdc.gov/std/

http://www.cdc.gov/hiv/prevention/research/prep/#

Chapter 12

~

Urinary Tract Infections

Anyone who has ever had to endure the itching, burning, and the constant feeling of the need to urinate caused by a urinary tract infection (UTI) can tell you that it is one of the most disruptive illnesses they have ever had. That body area has more nerve endings than any other area; it is not a good site to have invaded by bacteria causing inflammation. The illness can be as simple as a bladder infection, but can progress rapidly in some people to involve the kidney and possibly bloodstream infections. Having seen thousands of these patients end up in the hospital, I will give you some information that will help prevent these infections.

Urinary tract infections are particularly common in women, especially post-menopausal women. The urethra, the tube which carries urine from the bladder to the outside skin, is shorter in women than in men and, as women age, lower estrogen levels cause the skin to thin, allowing bacteria to reach the bladder from the outside skin more easily. This, coupled with a variety of reasons for incomplete bladder emptying, contributes to increased urinary tract infections in post-menopausal women. In addition to this, older men are at risk for urinary tract infections, especially prostate infections for various but similar reasons. During certain surgical procedures and hospital stays, patients have Foley catheters placed into the urethra and ending in the bladder. Because these catheters increase the risk of UTI, there is a concerted effort at hospitals to decrease the use of the catheters, mainly because Medicare has decreased payments to hospitals if there is a catheter related UTI during that hospital stay.

Urinary tract infections cannot completely be prevented due to the proximity of the bladder to outside skin where there are billions of bacteria. Certain bacteria such as *E. coli* have special properties that allow them to stick to bladder cells and cause infection. *E. coli* and other intestinal bacteria are at high concentrations in the groin area, even with the best hygiene practices. In obese patients, this is especially true due to difficulty with hygiene, extra skin folds, and excess moisture. A common question I am queried is, "Why did I get this infection? I am very clean around my house and I shower every day…"

I am also asked frequently, "How did I get *E. coli*?" The patient is thinking about the food poisoning strain of *E. coli* and she is now wondering what she ate that caused her to get this UTI. However, the strains that cause UTIs and food poisoning or traveler's diarrhea are different. Some strains have more of a capability to cause urinary tract infections and they are not the ones that cause diarrhea. We all have the bacteria called *E. coli* in our intestines that are usually benign. This bacterium is normally present in high numbers in the groin area. Their presence on the skin generally has nothing to do with bad hygiene.

It is not cleanliness that is the answer, it is the structural or flow issues that are the problem, which requires a completely different solution. Probably every young woman has heard the direction from their mother, "Make sure you empty your bladder after sexual relations, so you can prevent a urinary tract infection!!" This uncomfortable advice heard during young adulthood is partially true. Everything that will help prevent urinary infections has to do with keeping an empty bladder and keeping the flow going one direction and that is away from the kidneys and away from the bladder, out of the body. And it is not just true after sex!

The problems with this flow could be from a weak bladder muscle or an overactive bladder muscle. There could be structural problems associated with previous surgeries such as C-sections or other pelvic surgeries, childbirth, or prostate enlargement. Ureteroceles, prolapsed uterus, cystoceles, and rectoceles are prolapses of the ureter, uterus, bladder and the rectum that can alter the flow of urine. A prolapse occurs when the suspension or support of the organ fails and the organ protrudes into and may block other orifices. The urethra could be blocked partially, creating a flow issue.

If the flow issue is not due to a mechanical issue above, there are medications that can help with decreased urinary flow, depending on whether it is due to a weak bladder muscle or an enlarged prostate. Optimizing these medications can be achieved by your primary care physician or a Urologist. A urologist can perform a urinary flow test that will diagnose the problem. There are also procedures that may help but exercise caution about implanting devices when there is an ongoing infection.

With age, the skin around the urethra becomes thin because of lack of estrogen. This can be remedied by taking estrogen replacement therapy. There are risks associated with this therapy that have decreased its use; there is another option by using topical estrogen creams. The cream should be used liberally around the area of the urethra and the skin surrounding it. This will thicken the skin and perhaps decrease the ability for bacteria to travel up the urethra to the bladder. This should be the requisite therapy for all older women with frequent urinary tract infections.

Decreasing weight could help to limit pressure on the bladder and promote a stronger bladder. Some types of urinary retention and urinary incontinence may be improved after weight loss. In addition, good blood sugar control in diabetics could decrease the amount of sugar spilled into the urine, which could provide food for the bacteria. Even for nondiabetics, eliminating sugar intake may also help reduce bacterial growth in the bladder. There are some who espouse a special diet for people with frequent UTIs.

If kidney or bladder stones are present, bacteria inside the stone could be the problem, and it is possible the recurrences will not stop until the bacteria are killed or the stones are eliminated. Sometimes a stone will harbor bacteria within the stone making it harder to eliminate the bacteria. In this situation, the UTI causative organism is always the same organism found in the stone. If the bacteria found on culture are different each time then the stone is unlikely to be harboring multiple bacteria. Another reason kidney stones predispose one to infections is that kidney stones often cause microscopic bleeding which could provide food for the bacteria colonizing the bladder. In addition, if the stone disrupts the flow of urine, the bacteria may be more likely to ascend to the level of the kidney. A urologist should evaluate for the type of stones present because diets or medications can sometimes be used to eliminate the stones or prevent the stones from forming in the first place. See the information at the end of the chapter because a diet low in animal protein or a supplement of citric acid (or lemons or limes) could help.

It seems logical enough. Since we use antibiotics to treat UTI's why not try to prevent them with longer courses of antibiotics. Urologists for years have tried using antibiotics long term to prevent urinary tract infections. Because the bacteria in the intestines and the skin of the individuals treated with long-term antibiotics become resistant to the antibiotic used, this treatment is generally not effective for long. In addition, there are possible side effects of long-term antibiotic use. One potential area where this might be effective in the medium term is if a bacterium is being harbored in a small kidney stone.

An approach to make the bladder inhospitable to most bacteria could be the answer. There are many techniques to decreasing bacterial growth in the urinary system. Some involve making the urine more acidic, but this is not without controversy as one study showed a higher pH or less acidic urine could be the answer. Vitamin C and cranberry juice or cranberry tablets decrease the urinary pH, making bacterial growth less vigorous. Cranberry juice contains a compound called D-mannose that can inhibit attachment of bacteria to the bladder wall. Make sure you drink 100% cranberry juice and beware of cranberry "cocktail" that contains less juice and therefore less D-mannose, or ones with added sugar or high fructose corn syrup. There are over the counter D-mannose tablets available. Drinking lemon juice can give you Vitamin C and citric acid, which may be a double assault on urinary tract infections.

If you have kidney stones, be aware that increasing or decreasing your urine pH could predispose you to more kidney stones. Uric acid stones are more likely to form with more acidic urine and other stones are more likely with more alkaline (higher pH) urine. If you have had kidney stones in the past, ask your urologist before trying the above recommendations.

There are other compounds that are available by prescription such as methylene blue and methenamine hippurate that can also decrease bacterial growth in the urine. These methods are not guaranteed to decrease the frequency of UTI, but they have few side effects so they are an easy choice. For most persons with frequent urinary tract infections, the infections are not eliminated, but they are decreased. In my experience people who have 6 infections per year may have only 4. This is a godsend to some people.

Those with Foley catheters or suprapubic catheters are at increased risk of UTIs and there are more technical recommendations for prevention. A suprapubic catheter is a surgically implanted catheter directly into the bladder through the skin of the lower abdomen and is used when someone will need a catheter permanently. Prevention is centered on the sterility at insertion and prevention of bacteria climbing from outside the body into the bladder. This can happen inside the catheter or along the outside of the catheter. The concept of flow that we talked about above is key for this aspect.

Foley catheters should only be used if absolutely necessary; there are programs at hospitals now to decide this. In addition, there are more expensive Foley catheters that are lined with a silver or antibiotic compound. These catheters are less likely to become infected than the less expensive ones. If you are shopping for your own catheters through a medical supply store, make sure you get a quality catheter that has either of these compounds.

At insertion, until the catheter is fully inserted, it needs to be considered to be a sterile object and should touch nothing outside the sterile kit. Everything inside the kit is sterile (devoid of any bacteria or viruses). If the person inserting the catheter touches anything inside the kit with nonsterile gloves it is no longer sterile. The instructions in the catheter kit need to be followed to a "T". After cleaning the area where the catheter will be inserted (the urethra) with soap included in the kit, everything from that point onward should be sterile. Sterile gloves will be put on. The urethra will then be cleaned with an antiseptic swab, starting from the opening and, in circles, work outward from there, never inward toward the urethra. While both sterile gloves will be sterile at the start, once the nurse starts to touch other things outside the kit, only one hand should be used to touch these things. One hand should always remain sterile and that hand is the hand that is holding the Foley catheter. For example, if in a male patient, often the left hand is used to hold the penis and, even though this was cleaned, this hand will no longer be sterile and should not touch anything sterile (especially the catheter) until the catheter is fully inserted. There are classes and competencies that nurses and anyone else inserting the catheter should go through periodically in order to be qualified for inserting catheters.

Some surveys of the technique of Foley insertion show that only 30-60% of catheters were initially inserted completely correctly. Even the first step, putting on the gloves correctly shows only about an 80% correct technique. You could familiarize yourself with the directions for insertion and monitor this, but at a minimum the maintenance of sterility during the procedure is the most important part.

After insertion, an incredibly important concept will be not allowing anything inside the catheter and keeping the area where the catheter enters the body clean. The catheter system should not be disconnected unless absolutely necessary. The catheter bag should be drained often and should not fill beyond halfway full. After drainage, the drain at the bottom of the bag should be wiped with an alcohol wipe. The catheter bag should always be below the level of the bladder and hung as low as possible but should not lie on the floor.

There is another concept of dependent loops in a catheter's tubing. A dependent loop is formed when the tube of the catheter collection system hangs down and there is a "U" shape formed with the catheter exiting the body pointed downward (descending) and then going upward (ascending) and in certain catheters the tube has to point downward again to get into the bag. Urine collects in this loop creating pressure backwards into the bladder and could prevent emptying. To correct this, first the ascending part of the tube should be as short as possible, and, in general, the whole loop height should be as small as possible. One way to do this would be to increase the distance from the patient to the bag so that there is a long sloping descent and ascent. In other words, the bag should be at the foot of the bed if possible and if the patient has a leg bag (a bag that is attached to the leg) it should be attached lower if possible.

In hospital settings, the average percentage of Foley catheters without dependent loops ranges from 0-20%. I would imagine that at home, this percentage would be lower due to lack of education. Even in the hospital, there is a lack of education even though there is more and more information about dependent loops. This could impact your risk of infection, so if you have a Foley or suprapubic catheter, monitor this closely.

In addition, Foley catheters and suprapubic catheters need to be changed. How often it is changed will depend on individual circumstances and is decided by your urologist. Similar to the above notes regarding insertion, when a catheter is changed, it is paramount that sterile technique is followed. Foley catheters also need to be removed if no longer necessary as soon as it is feasible and advised by your physician.

You can see from the above information that a better diet and supplements can help protect you from the pain of frequent urinary tract infections. Remember the concept of flow and this will help you remember the concepts. The modern diet with high sugar intake may facilitate infection and can be corrected. Now, it is up to you, armed with this information, to make a conscious change in your diet, which may be easier said than done. Our modern society is accustomed to its sweets and this is a major obstacle to conquer. Reducing your risk of UTI will involve a close relationship between you and your urologist to keep the flow going and keep residual urine in the bladder to a minimum.

For more information:

Prevention of kidney stones:

http://www.mayoclinic.org/diseases-conditions/kidney-stones/basics/prevention/con-20024829

https://www.kidney.org/atoz/content/diet

Diet:

http://time.com/3941807/diet-uti-cranberry/

Dependent Loops:

https://vam.anest.ufl.edu/posters/Schwab2011.pdf

Chapter 13

~

Central Line, PICC Line, and Port Infections

In hospitals they are known as the dreaded abbreviation CLABSI, because they will soon result in decreased Medicare payment to the hospitals and the data for the infection rates for all hospitals are already published on public websites. Central Line Associated Bloodstream Infections are extremely common in the hospital, but can also occur at your home. Because of the frequent use of these central lines in the hospital, nursing facilities, and home, there has been an increase in the complications associated with them. The main complications are infections and blood clots. At least 2% of lines will have an infection (bacteria in the bloodstream or CLABSI) associated with them, which equates to 30,000 CLABSI per year or 80 line infections every day.

To illustrate the point, I was working in a clinic and saw an HIV patient for the first time and she told me she was being treated by a doctor in another county in an infusion center with daily IV azithromycin for a cough that she had. She had received about 7 days at that point and was telling me about fever and chills that had started the day before, just after her infusion. She had relatively stable lab tests according to her history. I promptly removed the PICC (peripherally inserted central catheter) line that she had in her arm and cultured the tip. In addition, we admitted her into the hospital for further IV antibiotics and she ended up having a PICC line associated bloodstream infection. (Of note, it is not appropriate to give intravenous antibiotics for bronchitis, especially azithromycin, which gets appropriate blood levels by pill form). A less egregious and more common example was a young lady receiving chemotherapy through a port who also had fevers. She was admitted to the hospital and also required intravenous antibiotics for a line infection. In general it is uncommon for someone to die of these infections, but it does occur and every time I see an infection, I try to assess if there was any way it could have been prevented.

Non-tunneled catheters such as triple lumen central lines are usually only used in hospitals but occasionally I have seen patients sent home with them. These are less safe at home because they are frequently associated with infections if left in for longer than 2 weeks. They are usually placed in the neck (jugular vein), upper chest (subclavian), or in the groin (femoral) and have three lumens or ports that merge into a single catheter at the entrance site. The safest site for most catheters is the subclavian (below the clavicle in the upper chest) area because there is less bacteria on the skin in this area and the area is easier to keep clean.

Tunneled central lines, such as Groshong and Hickman catheters are placed in the upper chest, travel under the skin to a large vein, and are slightly safer outside of the hospital. These catheters exit the skin and usually have one or two lumens or ports on the catheter. A port is also in the upper chest but unlike a Groshong or Hickman catheter, it is completely under the skin and a needle must be inserted into the skin and into the port to gain access.

A PICC line is also safer because it is tunneled. It enters a smaller vein in the bicep area therefore bacteria are slightly less likely to invade here. While a PICC line enters the vein in the arm its tip is in a large vein near the heart like all other catheters. Dialysis lines are larger catheters for hemodialysis that are either tunneled or non-tunneled (also called temporary). Temporary hemodialysis catheters can also be placed in the jugular, subclavian, or femoral sites. Tunneled hemodialysis catheters are less likely to become infected.

There are two types of infection, a tunnel infection and a bloodstream infection without tunnel infection. The first involves an infection around the outside of the catheter as it tunnels under the skin toward the vein. There is usually redness of the skin along that tunnel. In general it only occurs tunneled catheters such as ports, Groshong and Hickman catheters, or tunneled hemodialysis catheters. There can be fever, drainage, or bacteremia (bacteria growing in cultures of the blood). The most common symptom of bacteremia is fever and chills. If a line is infected and there is only fever or chills without the presence of redness, this could be a bloodstream infection without the tunnel infection. Both of these scenarios would indicate a CLABSI noted above. The potential end result could be a lengthy hospital stay, further antibiotics, and sepsis. Sepsis is an overwhelming infection that can be life threatening and can occur quickly. For this reason any fever while you have a line in place should be investigated with cultures.

Because of the increased rate of infections many hospitals adopted some safe practices when placing and caring for central lines. First, all lines should be placed using sterile practices. There are now checklists in hospitals to ensure a standard compliance with a bundle of safe practices to maintain a sterile field with no contaminants. Another best practice is to use a disk embedded with chlorhexidine soap over the line entrance site to prevent bacteria from colonizing this area. Each time a dressing is changed a similar sterile field should be maintained. After removing the old dressing, the area is cleaned with chlorhexidine. Then a new disk containing chlorhexidine should be placed over the entrance site. A clear, adherent, plastic dressing secures this in place, preventing soilage from the outside.

There has been an increase in the last 30 years in the use and overuse of these lines because of chemotherapy and other medications (including antibiotics) being infused through them. I have seen patients with ports in place because of frequent blood draws. This is not exactly the intended use of a port and is a potential recipe for disaster. In hospitals, it seems, everyone who is having difficulty with peripheral IV lines is having a central line placed, especially a PICC line because it is relatively easy to have a trained nurse place it. The other lines above require a physician to perform the procedure and therefore it is more difficult to obtain. There are, however, many appropriate reasons to have central lines and some rather simple steps can help prevent infections.

Similar to other infections it is useful to think of your skin as a cesspool of bacteria that are looking for the right place and time to invade. Having any type of central line provides those bacteria with direct access to the food that it wants, which is under your skin or in your bloodstream. Therefore the entrance site needs to be kept clean and dry and should be cared for exquisitely. Make sure that whoever places the line has placed a chlorhexidine disc at the entrance site as it has been shown to decrease infections. There will be a clear adhesive dressing (one brand name is Tegaderm) over the entrance site. This dressing should remain adherent to the skin so that no air or liquid can reach the entrance site. If the area will become wet such as in a shower, an additional layer of clear barrier can be used such as clear food wrap. The wrap should cover the catheter as well as the Tegaderm dressing making sure that neither of these becomes wet.

All persons accessing the ports of all central lines should sanitize their hands and use gloves to touch the ports. Before attaching the syringe or connecting tubing, both ends should be cleaned, usually with an alcohol or chlorhexidine swab. For some catheters there is an additional needle-less connector that prevents contamination of the inside of the line. These connectors should be changed periodically but usually not more often than every 72 hours. Dressing changes should be done at least weekly or more often if the area is soiled or if the dressing starts to peel away from the skin. Again the person doing the dressing change should use a mask and the patient should also wear a mask during the change. Once the clear dressing is removed the entrance site and the catheter hub should be cleaned with a chlorhexidine swab with the site allowed to dry before proceeding, because part of the bacterial killing effect of chlorhexidine is the alcohol in the liquid which needs to dry to kill the bacteria. A new chlorhexidine disc is placed and the new clear dressing is applied. There may be other protocols that can be used that use similar antiseptic solutions.

An antibiotic lock is a technique that places an antibiotic plus heparin in the lumens of the catheter instead of heparin alone and leaving it there until the next time the catheter is accessed. This technique usually uses vancomycin, vancomycin and ciprofloxacin, or vancomycin and ceftazidime antibiotics. Using the antibiotic lock technique to prevent infections resulted in a significant decrease in CLABSIs. Despite the findings, it is rarely done except in instances of port infections to help treat the infection without removing the port since once a port becomes infected it usually needs to be removed. If it cannot be removed for some reason, the risk of recurrence is high, and antibiotic locks have been an adjunct to prevent recurrence in these cases. Even in my own practice, I do not use this technique for prevention as it could result in increased resistance to antibiotics. It may have its place in certain patients who are immunocompromised, however.

Ports are a special circumstance because they are usually left in place for a longer period of time. Sometimes they are kept in place even when there is no valid reason to keep it there. This is a risk for the same reason that having an artificial joint continues to have a risk of infection long after surgery. It is not uncommon to have bacteria find their way into the bloodstream from the teeth or intestines. If bacteria are caught early by the immune system, then all is well. However, if there is a foreign device such as a port, the bacteria could stick to it prior to the immune system cell digesting it. The other method of infection of long-term indwelling ports would be through the lumen, as the port still has to be accessed for flushing periodically. Each time it is accessed, there is a chance a bacteria from the surface of the skin could enter into the port when the needle pokes through the skin.

Similar to other lines, the skin over the port should be scrubbed with chlorhexidine (and allowed to dry) prior to accessing and if a Huber needle (a needle that is bent 90 degrees specially made for ports) is going to be left in place for more than a few hours, then a chlorhexidine disk should be placed under the dressing. The dressing and needle should be changed at least every 7 days or with visible evidence of soiling or dressing non-adherence to the skin. Similar to PICC lines, the area needs to be protected with an extra layer of plastic wrap if the port is still accessed and the patient needs to be bathed. Care should be exercised to prevent soiling from above with saliva or wound drainage.

Once it is no longer needed, make sure to ask to have the port (or any other central catheter) evaluated for removal. The worst possible infection is from a port or line that is no longer necessary. Removal of most catheters is easier than the process of inserting them. If you need another line in the future, it can be reinserted.

In summary, to protect yourself from central line infections or CLABSIs, the most important thing is to be vigilant about the care and cleanliness around the entry site of the catheter. New chlorhexidine disks should be placed at every weekly dressing change. If the dressing becomes wet or soiled, it should be changed immediately. If the line becomes partially dislodged, the entire catheter needs to be changed. Hand washing and use of gloves at every handling of the ports and any tubing is an absolute necessity and the connectors should be wiped with an alcohol or chlorhexidine swab prior to connecting.

For More Information:

https://www.cdc.gov/hicpac/pdf/guidelines/bsi-guidelines-2011.pdf

Chapter 14

~

Chemotherapy and Monoclonal Antibody Related Infections

One thing that sets people whose immune system is impaired apart from everyone else is that the infections they get are worse than other people's infections and they could have different appearances from everyone else's infection. Even a simple cold sore that one person gets from herpes simplex can, in the patient after chemotherapy or monoclonal antibodies, cause ulcerations through the whole mouth and in the swallowing tube, the esophagus. We have seen a few patients who have had monoclonal antibodies, like infliximab (Remicade) or adalimumab (Humira), who have had a very difficult to treat form of meningitis, that we are still treating today.

The two topics of this chapter are like night and day. The infections patients may encounter because of these different immune suppressing drugs and the precautions one must take are very different. Chemotherapy is becoming less toxic as more specific targeting of cancer cells is discovered; however, the number one killer of cancer patients remains infection. The highest rates of infection have always been with chemotherapy for leukemias and lymphomas. Chemotherapy for these cancers of the blood and lymphatic system must target the very immune system that produces the cancer cells. Most chemotherapy causes the immune system to be knocked out (producing a condition of very low numbers of neutrophils – infection fighting cells - called neutropenia) for a longer period of time with these treatments, thus higher rates of infection. Treatments of other cancers continue to present problems with neutropenia (a low number of infection fighting white blood cells), albeit less commonly than in the past, and infections remain one of the top complications. Bone marrow and stem cell transplants present unique complications because not only are neutrophils targeted, but other kinds of infection-fighting cells called T cells are also impaired. Newer monoclonal antibody treatments are available for cancers and many other diseases such as rheumatoid arthritis, asthma, and Crohn's disease and they manifest with other types of infections. You can tell a medication is a monoclonal antibody because the generic name ends in "mab" like the above infliximab. The infections with these medications vary from tuberculosis to viral infections, which is much different from traditional chemotherapy.

We will tackle the worst first. As mentioned above, leukemias and lymphomas are cancers of the blood and lymphatic system. There are acute (suddenly appearing) and chronic (lasting for long periods of time) leukemias. The chronic leukemias are more indolent in that they are slow growing and often have few symptoms until late in the disease. Likewise, the treatments are less toxic and there are some newer oral chemotherapy treatments available that have less infectious complications but introduce their own problems. Acute leukemias however, have quick onsets, higher mortality, and significant symptoms. The leukemia cells overtake normal bone marrow cells, producing anemia and fatigue, low platelet counts with bleeding, and low numbers of effective infection fighting cells with resultant infections. To every leukemia patient it seems counterintuitive. The white blood cell (WBC) count is high and therefore one would think these infection fighting cells would be effective at fighting infection, but they are not since they are abnormal and function poorly. Functionally, this puts them at increased risk for more dangerous infections.

Let's step back and talk about the immune system. There are white blood cells that have different functions, comprised of lymphocytes, phagocytes, and neutrophils. Lymphocytes are comprised of B cells and T cells. B cells produce antibodies that recognize foreign agents such as viruses and bacteria. Once the antibody attaches to an invader, phagocytes or T cells kill the bacteria or ingest the virus to hopefully inactivate it. T cells also kill fungi and certain parasites. The neutrophils are present in the bloodstream and are activated in bacterial and fungal infections to ingest and kill these types of invaders.

When patients have problems with antibodies, they may experience frequent bacterial infections. When there are problems with T cells, fungal, parasitic, and viral infections such as those seen with AIDS patients may develop. Neutropenia involves a low neutrophil count and any number of infections occur depending on the duration of the neutropenia. A patient with neutropenia for a week or less is at risk for invasion of gut bacteria and viruses. After a week, skin and mouth bacteria and fungi also invade. After two weeks, there are other fungi and mold and other viruses that can raise their ugly head. The molds that invade have been the most fatal infections but now we more recently have better antifungal medications approved to treat them.

During the first phase, in the first week of neutropenia, fever is common. Sixty percent of the time no recognizable infection is found and when the neutropenia resolves, the fever dissipates. The billions of bacteria in the intestines may be involved or it could also be the myriad of viruses already present in the body that may be causative in these cases where no infection is found. In addition, there could be no infection at all, and fever could be a side effect of the chemotherapy or of the process of killing the cancer cells called tumor necrosis. When infection is found, it is often pneumonia or central line/port infections. Ports or other central venous lines are present to allow the chemotherapy to be administered and accessing these ports puts them at risk for infection. *Staphylococcus* predominates, but other gut bacteria as well as fungi, can cause port infections. See also the chapter on ports and central lines.

During the second phase from 7 to 14 days, there are other infections that relate to the longer duration of neutropenia. This longer duration allows bacteria from the intestines more time to cross the intestinal barriers and invade into the bowel wall causing a condition called typhlitis. Because there are higher concentrations of bacteria in the right side of the colon, this condition produces right-sided abdominal pain. Fungal infections become more common due to central venous lines and also the intestinal fungi that are present. Toward the end of this immune-suppressed period and later, viruses start to cause infections. Cytomegalovirus, BK virus, Epstein-Barr virus, and adenovirus are common.

From 14 days onward, any opportunistic bug can invade, including the above-mentioned ones. We especially see mold infections such as *Aspergillus, Fusarium,* and *Scedosporium* in this time period. These critters especially like to invade our bodies via inhalation and direct inoculation of the skin. Everyone has some amount of mold on their feet due to the moist areas of the shoes we wear and common mold infections that we may already have, referred to as athlete's foot. We ingest molds every time we eat allowing the GI tract also to be a possible site of invasion. Uncooked foods, especially fruits and vegetables, have molds on their surfaces. The ingestion of antibiotics that are given to prevent infection, may select for resistant bacteria, fungi, and molds as the predominant organisms in the intestines. For this reason, antifungal agents are often given to prevent these infections in certain patients expected to have more prolonged neutropenia.

Monoclonal antibody treatments are being used for a wide variety of illnesses now. These treatments target the cells that are causing the illness whether they may be your own cells or cancer cells or invading cells. The illnesses vary from asthma, rheumatoid arthritis and Crohn's disease to cancers and leukemias. The treatments cause a small decrease in the immune system that puts one at risk for many infections. The increase in risk usually does not require a mention other than three infections: tuberculosis, histoplasmosis, and hepatitis, though there are other infections that occur.

Infliximab (Remicade), adalimumab (Humira), etanercept (Enbrel), and certolizumab (Cimzia) are all tumor necrosis factor (TNF) inhibitors. TNF (a chemical signal protein) alerts different immune system cells that there is inflammation or infection. It is one of the primary causes of fever and can inhibit virus and tumor growth. Blocking TNF can inhibit inflammation in different areas of the body and have been used to treat inflammatory conditions such as rheumatoid arthritis and Crohn's disease.

Persons who are treated with the TNF blockers listed above are at risk for viral infections. Hepatitis B and C could increase replication while on these medications. It is well known that while on immunosuppressants that especially Hepatitis B could flare causing more liver inflammation and destruction. Some of the patients on TNF blockers were on other immunosuppressants at the same time making it unclear which had the biggest impact. In addition, cytomegalovirus, herpes simplex viruses, varicella-zoster virus (shingles), Epstein-Barr virus, and other viruses could cause a viral syndrome with rashes while on these medications.

Granulomatous diseases are increased in patients on TNF blockers. The main infection risks, Tuberculosis (TB) and histoplasmosis are reported to be increased in these patients. Of the first 170,000 persons treated with Remicade, there were about 80 cases of serious life-threatening TB. If there is a latent infection with TB in the lungs (see the chapter on TB), the blocking of TNF may cause the body to lose immune control of the organism. Histoplasma is a fungus that is common in the Mississippi and Ohio River areas and is found in bird droppings and soil. It is controlled by the same type of mechanisms that wall off TB in the lungs. Other possible granulomatous infections include candidiasis (yeast skin infections), cryptococcosis (meningitis), coccidioidomycosis (lung infection and meningitis in Southwestern US), listeria (fever and meningitis after eating deli meats and cheeses), nocardiosis (skin, lung, and brain infection from soil or plant exposure), and atypical mycobacteria (cousins of TB causing skin and lung infections). TNF blockers also inhibit the immune response to non-granulomatous, intracellular bacteria such as Legionella that causes and atypical pneumonia after

To protect oneself from bacteria is like protecting your house from invasion by cockroaches. Bacteria are already present inside every orifice of your body, on your skin, and in your intestines, but there are other more invasive bacteria to be more worried about. Avoiding other people that are ill is the first step. There are a few experts who advocate using masks while in public, but most would say this is excessive. Avoiding undercooked foods and soft cheeses will help prevent food borne illnesses. Protect your port and maintain good clean hygiene of the skin around the port.

To protect oneself from tuberculosis, there are a few easy steps. Tuberculosis is more common in crowded places, such as jails, homeless shelters, and other crowded living facilities. It is also more common in other countries, so places where immigrants are congregating could present a risk. In general, you have to have prolonged close contact with a person with active TB to contract the illness. Healthcare workers are also at risk. The key to preventing TB lies in detecting the exposure early after it occurs. To do this, a skin test with purified protein derivative (PPD) or a blood test called Quantiferon Gold can detect the bacteria soon after it enters the body. This test should be done before you become immune suppressed (before starting any of the medications mentioned above) and

114

yearly thereafter. If positive, you should be treated for TB infection unless there are extenuating circumstances. Please also see the separate chapter on TB.

To protect oneself from viruses is the most difficult task. These viruses are already present in your body and they can and will reactivate. Detection of that reactivation is key, especially in the case of cytomegalovirus (CMV). Medications to prevent infection by CMV are given to certain patients usually bone marrow transplant patients and solid organ transplant patients and your physician determines this with blood tests. Other herpes viruses such as Herpes Simplex (HSV) and Epstein - Barr virus (EBV) also can cause infections. Medications to prevent HSV reactivation can be given during substantial chemotherapy regimens such as those for leukemia.

To protect one from molds, stay away from construction sites and places where there is dust in the air. Avoid birds and bird droppings, especially caves, trees, and anywhere else that bird droppings may be. Do not garden when your immune system is at its lowest. Wear gloves when handling soil and take extra precautions when gardening or if you will be in contact with vegetation. Flowers may have mold on their leaves and petals. Inhalation or the minutest skin break could present a point of invasion for the mold. Avoiding eating raw unpeeled vegetables and fruits with skins will also protect you from mold infections. Never walk barefoot, keep a close eye on your feet, and treat any athlete's foot that is present aggressively.

There are other monoclonal antibodies that may affect the immune system and therefore increase the risk of infection. One in particular affects the epidermal growth factor system and does not directly affect the immune system. However it may affect the lining of the mouth and intestines increasing the possibility of infections in these areas.

A note is inserted here about infusion therapies. Many forms of chemotherapy and monoclonal antibodies are infused intravenously. In addition, antbiotics, immunoglobulins, and other therapies are given to patients in this manner. There are alternative or homeopathic treatments such as chelation that are also performed on patients. Every year there are investigations regarding diseases such as hepatitis B and C that are transmitted to patients because of negligent techniques. For example, an investigation of a chelation center occurred where the nurse was using the same syringe that she had just flushed the IV, to obtain the medication from the shared vial. This introduced the virus into the vial, which was then spread to the other patients. Another egregious example happened when the doctor was doing infusions on himself after hours, and contaminated shared vials. These examples are outliers, but are also not uncommon enough for you not to be vigilant. If you are receiving any type of intravenous therapy, be sure to look for these types of practices. It is best to have patient specific vials, but multi-use vials are not uncommon and are safe if best practices are adhered to.

Thus there is a lot to think about with all of these treatments. Become as informed as you can about exposures that will put you at highest risk and avoid these at all costs. If this means giving up gardening or certain foods for a few weeks at a time just after chemotherapy or at all times during monoclonal antibody treatment, this is a small cost for saving your life because these infections are often so difficult to treat and if a mold infection occurs, the mortality is often high despite aggressive antifungal treatment.

Lastly, do some research on the guidelines for the use of preventive antibiotics and antivirals during certain chemotherapies. I have added guideline papers from oncology journals but by the time you read this, they may be out of date, so do your own research and discuss this with your physician. Many community oncologists and hospitals are not up to date on the guidelines. In general, as of the 2012 guidelines, if you are receiving chemotherapy that causes you to be neutropenic for longer than 7 days, if you are receiving higher dose corticosteroids such as prednisone, or if you have chronic active hepatitis B, you may benefit from preventive antibiotics. Chemotherapy for acute leukemias and some lymphomas and bone marrow transplants (hematopoietic stem cell transplants) often cause neutropenia for longer than 7 days and should be given preventive antibiotics, antifungals, and antivirals against herpes simplex.

For more information:

http://jco.ascopubs.org/content/31/6/794.full

Chapter 15

∽

Antibiotics

Antibiotics have been a godsend for the human race since penicillin was first discovered in the 1940s. In World War I, an astonishing number of soldiers were killed by infections. This includes the great influenza outbreak of 1918, but the infections, mostly bacterial, following gunshot wounds or other injuries outnumber those killed solely by the blasts themselves. By World War II and Korea, we started to change infection-related deaths due to the advent of sulfa and penicillin antibiotics. This is merely an example during wartime, but in civilian life the same could be said to be true. Routine injuries, car accidents, pneumonia, and childbirth over a few decades became more manageable for medical doctors due to antibiotics.

However, this is not without a cost, because the fascination with being able to cure infectious diseases turned into the overuse of antibiotics in the 1980s and 1990s. The unintended side effects from antibiotics have caused a myriad of significant problems including rashes, diarrhea, and other adverse events, sometimes resulting in death. In order to protect yourself from these effects, you need to be educated about possible side effects. If you are aware of the possible side effects, you can be better informed of the risks of taking them and perhaps be less likely to ask for antibiotics from your doctor. If you and your physician decide antibiotics are the right choice for you, you will also be more likely to recognize these known side effects earlier.

In this chapter, I will be going over just some of the common side effects or possible complications and warnings about antibiotics, either in general or specifically regarding a particular class of antibiotics. This is not an exhaustive list of possible antibiotic complications. What I want you to take away from this is to research the side effects and be aware of the possible side effects before you ask your doctor for antibiotics. Understanding there is a potential adverse cost that can alter the benefit of the prescription is clearly important.

Bacterial resistance to antibiotics has been occurring for the last 40 years and is getting worse. Over-prescribing antibiotics and agricultural use of antibiotics has created and magnified this problem. However, there is a misconception that I hear often from patients. It is usually a family member who asks, "But if my wife receives antibiotics, won't she be more susceptible to infections because the antibiotics will lower her immune system?" Antibiotics do not lower your resistance to infection; rather, the antibiotics could create resistant bacteria by inducing bacterial resistance in your intestines. These bacteria could create an infection that then is resistant to the normal antibiotics your doctor may prescribe for you. You do not become resistant to the antibiotics, the bacteria do.

The bacteria in your intestines share the resistance that they gain from exposure to antibiotics that you swallow. It is possible to share these same resistant bacteria with your family, friends and everyone else you are encounter. Later, if you or others come down with an infection, it may be more likely to be resistant to the usual antibiotics that you are prescribed.

Another way that antibiotics can have either minor or devastating effects is by killing benign bacteria in the intestines. Bacteria normally have wars against each other in the intestines; there are a host of benign bacteria that assist your intestines with digestion and promote overall health. Each bacteria keeps the next one suppressed to manageable levels. *Clostridium difficile* (C. diff) is a bacterium that is discussed in another chapter and will not be discussed much here, but if it is able to grow unchecked after antibiotics kill benign intestinal bacteria, a potentially deadly disease can ensue. The fluoroquinolone antibiotics (ciprofloxacin, levofloxacin, and moxifloxacin), cephalosporins (cephalexin, cefuroxime, ceftriaxone, etc.), and clindamycin are more likely than other antibiotics to cause C. diff infections, but all antibiotics can do so. If you have any diarrhea while on an antibiotic report it to your doctor. See additional information in the chapter on C. diff.

The following side effect and drug interaction information is just a partial list of side effects to watch for from certain antibiotics. This is not intended to be an exhaustive list and you should consult with your physician and pharmacist about possible side effects and drug interactions you may have. These are the more common side effects.

Penicillins and cephalosporins include amoxicillin, Augmentin, cephalexin, keflex, and ceftin. If the generic name starts with a cef- or ends in -cillin then it is in this class of medications. Rashes and diarrhea are common. Augmentin causes diarrhea so frequently we as doctors are usually prepared to prescribe probiotics to prevent it. Probiotics such as the bacteria in yogurt or the pill form called lactobacillus, acidophilus, or other names can help prevent the diarrhea caused by antibiotics as long as it is not caused by C. diff. Rarely there can be other side effects that can cause arthritis symptoms.

Macrolides include erythromycin, azithromycin, and clarithromycin. The gastrointestinal side effects of these antibiotics include nausea, epigastric pain, and diarrhea. Azithromycin can cause liver issues. These medications can increase a cardiac parameter called the QT interval that could lead to a fatal cardiac arrest. This is usually not an issue unless the antibiotic is coupled with another medication that prolongs the QT interval, including but not limited to amiodarone, Sotalol or some antifungal medications. When taking a macrolide it will be important to let your doctor and pharmacist know all of your medications including over the counter and supplements.

Quinolone antibiotics such as levofloxacin, ciprofloxacin, and moxifloxacin are often used for respiratory and urinary tract infections. At one point they were the most commonly prescribed antibiotics. They also increase the QT interval (especially levofloxacin and moxifloxacin) should not be prescribed with other QT prolonging drugs. They can also interfere with cartilage maintenance and have been associated with joint pain and tendon rupture. Achilles tendon rupture has occurred very commonly with these antibiotics. I tell patients on these antibiotics that they need to avoid putting stress on their Achilles tendon. It is prudent to avoid playing basketball and climbing ladders while on these antibiotics. In addition, when climbing stairs, the entire foot should be placed on each step, because dangling the heel over the edge of the step and placing the body's weight on the ball of the foot only places a lot of stress on the Achilles tendon.

I had a friend who was somewhat overweight and looked like someone who would never run or exercise. To the contrary he was a member of a competitive basketball team until he was prescribed a quinolone for a prostate infection for a 4 week course. In the middle of the course of antibiotics he played a game of basketball and suffered a debilitating Achilles tendon tear. This took him weeks to recover and he did not play basketball for months.

Avoid taking quinolone antibiotics within 2 hours before or after dairy products (which contain calcium), antacids (which contain calcium carbonate, aluminum hydroxide, or magnesium hydroxide), or iron containing vitamins or supplements. The effect of taking these at the same time is decreased absorption of the antibiotic; you can take these during the same day, just separate from the antibiotic by at least 2 hours. The antacids mentioned above that you need to avoid do not include acid blockers such as ranitidine (Zantac), famotidine (Pepcid), omeprazole, lansoprazole, and other similar medications.

Tetracyclines such as doxycycline and minocycline often have nausea and upset stomach as a side effect. They can also cause pancreatitis – a more severe upset stomach involving the pancreas. If you develop a severe headache while on a tetracycline consult your physician regarding a potentially serious side effect. A sunburn reaction to sunlight, also called a photosensitive rash can occur also. This is not an allergic reaction. Instead, sun exposure of the skin leads a more intense sunburn while on these types of antibiotics. If you are on this antibiotic, take precautions to avoid sun exposure or cover the skin with a hat and long sleeves and pants. I once had a patient who covered all of her skin but her hands but nonetheless she still sustained a moderately severe sunburn on her hand from being in the sun for 30 minutes driving her motorized scooter around the neighborhood. Similar to quinolones, avoid taking these antibiotics within 2 hours before or after antacids (Tums, Rolaids, etc.) that contain calcium, aluminum, or magnesium, multivitamins or other medications that contain iron, or dairy products. There will not be an adverse event, but the antibiotic may not be absorbed as well.

Sulfonamides are commonly referred to as sulfa antibiotics and include Bactrim and Septra. Allergic rash is very common, as is the photosensitive rash mentioned previously. Therefore, stay out of the sun if you are on a sulfa antibiotic. A far more serious and potentially deadly rash called Stevens Johnson syndrome can occur so report any start of a rash promptly to your doctor. Kidney damage can rarely occur while on sulfa drugs.

Nitrofurantoin and similar antibiotics are commonly used for urinary tract infections, and should not be used for any other type of infection. They can cause an allergic type of reaction often without a rash causing shortness of breath, wheezing, and cough, especially if used for longer than a few days. Often the only symptom is a cough and is called hypersensitivity pneumonitis. These antibiotics cannot be used if there is significant previous kidney damage because the antibiotic cannot make it into the urine if the kidneys are not working properly.

Metronidazole is an antibiotic that is used for a myriad of infections. It possesses a disulfiram reaction when the user imbibes alcohol. This disulfiram reaction will cause severe vomiting with even the smallest amount of alcohol ingestion. Even cough syrup that has some small amounts of alcohol could cause vomiting while the patient is on metronidazole. Therefore, do not drink any alcohol while on this medication.

The antibiotic linezolid that has precautions for interactions with certain antidepressants, fentanyl, and tramadol. Ask your doctor about drug interactions with this medication. The antibiotic also can cause anemia. The drug can also rarely cause nerve damage.

Vancomycin is a common antibiotic to be given in the hospital for staph infections. It can cause kidney issues and sometimes causes a rash, especially if it is infused too rapidly. Most times the rash is better or prevented if the infusion rate is slowed down. Rarely abdominal pain during the infusion of intravenous Vancomycin could occur. Vancomycin by mouth is only used for intestinal infections because it does not get absorbed and stays in the intestines where the offending bacteria are located.

Because of the above potentially serious side effects and the potential for development of resistance, only use antibiotics on the advice of a doctor. In addition, research the possible side effects of all of your medications. Understand the information on side effects may include symptoms that are unrelated to the medication, so ask your physician if your symptoms are due to the medication.

Above all, only use antibiotics as prescribed by your doctor and finish the full course unless you have significant side effects and are directed to stop by your doctor. Using previously prescribed antibiotics likely will not be the right one for your infection and implies that you did not appropriately finish the previous course. I have experienced hundreds of patients who have done potentially serious harm to themselves by self-prescribing their antibiotics.

If you have diarrhea while on an antibiotic it could be caused by *Clostridium difficile* diarrhea, which is the subject of another chapter. You should have your feces checked for this bacteria. If you do not have this, the antibiotic itself likely caused your diarrhea. This can be remedied by taking probiotics, which are the same bacteria that are in yogurt. If you do not like yogurt, there are companies that make a pill form of this bacteria. Many people take probiotics regularly to keep their intestines full of benign bacteria and many swear by their ability to keep them regular.

Be wise and leave the medical advice to your doctor. Make sure your doctor and pharmacist explain the benefits and side effects of all antibiotics you are prescribed. Contact the doctor or your pharmacist with any side effect you may be having as it could be significant, but also may have a relatively simple fix. Read the information that is attached to your prescription at the pharmacy. And don't forget to take probiotics if you are on antibiotics to prevent diarrhea and to promote beneficial digestion.

Chapter 16

~

Meningitis and Encephalitis

Meningitis is often thought of as a very deadly disease of young college aged adults. However, it can strike persons of any age and each age group has its own particular set of bacteria and viruses that cause this syndrome. About 4,000 cases of bacterial meningitis and 75,000 cases of viral meningitis occur in the US every year; however, 1.2 million cases of bacterial meningitis occur worldwide and 170,000 deaths occur worldwide. The yearly incidence of bacterial meningitis in the US has decreased by 75% over the past 3 decades, mostly because of pneumococcal and *Haemophilus* vaccinations. The devastating form of meningitis is caused by *Neisseria meningitidis*. Meningitis can also be caused by a myriad of bacteria, viruses, and fungi. Meningitis also can be caused by certain medications or autoimmune conditions such as rheumatoid arthritis or lupus.

The symptoms of meningitis include headache, stiff neck, fever, muscle aches, weakness, and lethargy. Photophobia is sensitivity to bright light and phonophobia is sensitivity to loud noises. A purple rash usually occurs with *Neisseria meningitidis* infection. Confusion and bizarre behavior can occur, especially with herpes simplex encephalitis. Loss of consciousness can occur early, and portends a bad outcome.

Encephalitis occurs when the organism infects the brain as opposed to just infecting the brain covering, hence the symptoms of unusual behavior and hallucinations. Viruses, especially herpes simplex and enteroviruses, usually cause encephalitis. Mosquito-borne viruses such as West Nile Virus, Eastern Equine Virus, and other similar viruses cause encephalitis especially occurring in more rural areas.

The most severe form of meningitis is caused by bacteria. In babies, group B streptococcus causes meningitis, but is uncommon now with treatment of group B strep colonization during pregnancy. *Haemophilus influenzae* previously was a major cause of childhood meningitis, but now with vaccinations it is very unusual. *Streptococcus pneumoniae* is the most common cause of meningitis in adults, but is far less common now, also because of vaccination use. *Neisseria meningitidis* causes a rapidly progressing illness that can be fatal in 24 hours, usually in young adults, and has been spread in close quarters such as college or military dormitories. *Listeria* is another bacteria that can cause meningitis in pregnant women, immune suppressed, and older adults.

Viral meningitis is less severe and is caused by a myriad of types of viruses. Even the common cold virus could cause meningitis, albeit relatively uncommonly. The enterovirus family of viruses causes many cases of viral meningitis. These illnesses are usually far less severe than those caused by bacteria and are common across all age groups. There is usually no treatment unless herpes simplex, varicella-zoster virus (the chickenpox or shingles virus) or cytomegalovirus is causing the disease.

Fungi can also cause meningitis, but almost exclusively in immune suppressed or post-neurosurgical patients. *Cryptococcus* is a known cause of meningitis in AIDS patients but we have seen it rarely in persons without immunosuppression. *Histoplasma* can cause meningitis in the Midwest while *Coccidioides* can cause meningitis in the Southwest.

So how can you protect yourself from this disastrous scourge? Most of the answer will rely on vaccinations, as you may have guessed; however, there are other things we can do. When I am seeing a case of viral meningitis, the first question that I get from family members (and nurses) is, "How do I prevent this from occurring to me after I have been exposed to my relative?" The answer is usually standard precautions of infection prevention – especially hand hygiene.

In cases of viral or so-called "aseptic" meningitis, your protection involves the same preventive measures that you would take with any viral infection. Usually the viruses involved are spread by respiratory, contact, or fecal route. Hand washing and managing exposure to fomites (secretions, feces, and urine) will be key. Both patient and caregiver should wash hands with an alcohol gel frequently. When handling clothing or sheets soiled with any secretions, gloves should be worn.

With that said, most cases of viral meningitis do not need to be strictly isolated. Since the virus involved may be the same virus as the common cold or "stomach flu", if the exposed person does contract the virus, the likelihood of it causing meningitis in them will be very low. It will more likely cause a common cold or "stomach flu" in any family members who become ill. It is exceedingly rare for more than one family member to be ill with viral meningitis at the same time.

Because of the severity and contagiousness of bacterial meningitis, it is more important to protect yourself from contracting it. As I stated before, the incidence of bacterial meningitis in the US has decreased by more than 75% and is less than 10% of the incidence in other countries due to a high vaccination rate for *Haemophilus, Streptococcus pneumoniae*, and *Neisseria meningitidis* in the at risk groups, as well as good prenatal care which includes screening for carriage of group B strep near the womb.

Only in cases of bacterial meningitis caused by *Neisseria meningitidis* is there any prevention available after exposure to someone with meningitis. If a loved one, or very close contact, has this bacteria causing meningitis, and it is still within 72 hours of the exposure, you should take an antibiotic to prevent yourself from contracting meningitis. Talk with your physician, immediately if possible as preventative effectiveness is believed to be best if taken within 72 hours after exposure. In healthcare workers, the exposure has to be a significant exposure to respiratory secretions before antibiotics are given. There is some data for taking a preventive antibiotic in *Haemophilus influenzae* meningitis but it is not often given. Vaccinations should also be given to family members of and exposures to patients with *Neisseria meningitidis* and *Haemophilius influenzae* meningitis.

Protecting newborns from meningitis involves screening for group B strep during pregnancy. This is routinely done during prenatal visits later in pregnancy, therefore, you usually do not need to monitor this. Premature neonates are at increased risk. You can be proactive with this and keep track of your lab tests at each visit. Most obstetricians have full protocols for all laboratory studies that are standard of care and with electronic medical records it is easy to access these labs.

To protect yourself from pneumococcal meningitis, vaccinations are important. Conjugate pneumococcal vaccines are given in childhood and you should keep up with this vaccine during your children's pediatrician office visits. Adult vaccinations with two separate vaccinations (a conjugate pneumococcal vaccine called Prevnar and a polysaccharide vaccine called Pneumovax) should be given if you are over 50 or at younger age if you have certain conditions that put you at risk for pneumonia. These are cirrhosis, congestive heart failure, diabetes mellitus, sickle cell disease (or other lack of a functional spleen), chronic renal failure, and patients with certain cancers.

Because *Neisseria meningitidis* primarily impacts young adults 16 to 25 years of age, the immunization recommendations are geared toward pediatricians vaccinating at age 16 or prior to heading off to college. In addition, travel recommendations include vaccinating prior to travel to Northern Africa or to the Hajj in Mecca, Saudi Arabia. There are now two types of vaccines available and both are recommended. For years we have had a vaccine covering 4 of the 12 serotypes of Neisseria meningitidis. There is a fifth serotype, Serotype B that has not been covered in the past due to difficulty in creating a vaccine for this type. The importance of this serotype in the US is paramount because historically it has been the third most common serotype, and quickly is becoming the most common type of epidemic on college campus. In 2015, 2 vaccines were approved for Serotype B. It is now recommended to give both vaccines to the above at risk individuals.

Thus, it is relatively easy to protect yourself from bacterial meningitis. To protect yourself from viral meningitis involves actions you already perform in your daily lives. Remember that protecting yourself also involves being proactive in your care because some physicians do not routinely consider giving some of these vaccinations mentioned throughout this book.

Chapter 17

~

Naegleria fowleri and Primary Amoebic Meningoencephalitis

As a nod to a dear colleague of mine, this chapter is dedicated to her 10-year-old son whom she lost to the "brain eating" amoeba called *Naegleria fowleri* in 2009. *Naegleria* (along with many other amoebae) exists in warm, fresh waters, especially in the summer time. Lakes, ponds and streams can harbor this parasite. It is usually stirred up from the bottom sediment in shallow water. With global warming, the temperature of waters is increasing and what previously was thought to be a problem only in Florida has been found as far north as Minnesota. Unsuspecting young people have contracted this disease from dunking their head under the water in water activities such as swimming, tubing, or skiing.

In addition, outdoor hoses and "slip and slides" have been implicated. Tap water not only has bacteria but also could have the parasites present, especially if chlorination levels are low. Primary amoebic meningoencephalitis (PAM) has also been found to be caused by non-sterile nasal rinses, using neti pots that help to clear nasal passages. If tap water that is not sterilized by boiling is used in these rinses, then the amoeba could persist and be instilled into the nasal cavities, causing this devastating disease. Any pool that uses inadequately chlorinated water could also put you at risk.

The problem with watersports and swimming arises when the water warms to the temperatures of summertime. Above 80 degrees Fahrenheit, the parasite grows very well. When instilled into the nasal cavity, the para-

127

site can begin to invade through the sinuses and then into the brain. From 1962 to 2008 approximately 111 documented cases of primary amoebic meningoencephalitis have occurred in the US. In 2007-2008, 8 fatalities unfortunately occurred. The numbers are likely higher and are seeming to increase every year, since it is difficult to diagnose. Worldwide cases are often undiagnosed but probably more common than in the US due to swimming in sewage infested rivers and certain religious practices such as ablution.

The mortality from primary amoebic meningoencephalitis is at least 95% owing to late diagnosis, a lack of effective antibiotics, and the aggressiveness of the infection. Better awareness in the medical community has helped to diagnose victims earlier. Groups such as Amoebaseason. com are educating the public and medical community. There is a new experimental treatment that is recently approved to treat this devastating disease. The medication, miltefosine, has shown promise in decreasing the mortality, especially if given early in the disease. There have been a few survivors over the past year, which is remarkable.

To protect yourself from this parasite, avoid dunking your head underwater when swimming in warm waters. If this is unavoidable, you must use a simple nose clip, often used by competitive swimmers, which prevents nasal water entry. It is recommended for all water activities in these warm waters. During all water sports such as waterskiing and tubing, always wear a nose clip. When using a neti pot and similar nasal rinses, boil the water and sanitize the container (then obviously let it cool to a safe temperature while in the container) prior to instilling the solution into the nose. Only use chlorinated water when using "bouncy houses" and "slip and slides" that have a water source and, again, nose clips should be worn.

By all means have fun in the water in the summer but be educated about the danger lurking in the warm waters and tell your friends. The life you save likely will be one that has a long life ahead of him or her.

For more information:

http://web.stanford.edu/group/parasites/ParaSites2010/Katherine_
Fero/FeroNaegleriafowleri.htm

Hlavsa MC, Roberts VA, Anderson AR, Hill VR, Kahler AM, Orr M, Garrison LE, Hicks LA, Newton A, Hilborn ED, Wade TJ, Beach MJ, Yoder JS. Surveillance for waterborne disease outbreaks and other health events associated with recreational water use — United States, 2007–2008. MMWR Surveill Summ. 2011;60:1-37.

Yoder JS, Eddy BA, Visvesvara GS, Capewell L, Beach MJ. The epidemiology of primary amoebic meningoencephalitis in the USA, 1962-2008. External Web Site Icon Epidemiol Infect. 2010;138:968-75.

http://www.Amoeba-Season.com

Chapter 18

~

Eye Infections

The amazing human eye can resist infections unlike any other organ in the body. Every day the eye pumps tears by blinking from tear glands located in the outer corner across the eye to ducts that carry them from the inner corner into the nasal cavity. Within these tears there are substances that help protect the eye from hostile invaders. The glands and ducts are very tiny, intricate pieces of anatomy. So too are the parts of the inner eye, and this part of the eye has a thick defense shield to keep all germs out. However, when infection goes wrong here, it goes REALLY wrong!! Once inside the eyeball, the defenses are minimal and infection is difficult to treat.

I have seen devastating infections of the inner eye called endophthalmitis caused by fungi and bacteria whose appearance would make a person with a strong constitution lose their lunch. Some of these infections come from within our body and are carried from a distant site through the bloodstream, but mostly they are from local spread of invasive organisms. From the unfortunate soul who was unlucky enough to get a post-surgical infection after a cataract surgery to the contact wearer who did not follow the directions of the eye doctor, these infections can be devastating when one loses sight from them.

Contact lens wearers are acutely aware of the dangers to their eyes. It is an unusual contact lens wearer who has not had some sort of pink eye from wearing contacts. The solutions that contact wearers use to clean their contacts have preservatives to prevent growth of bacteria, but absolute care needs to be taken with the whole process. It is important not to touch the tip of the bottle to anything including fingers, contact case, and towels, because doing so will allow bacteria or fungi to enter the bottle. It is essential to wash your hands with soap and water before touching your eye or any of the equipment. Similarly the cases that are used to disinfect contacts need to be cleaned and rinsed frequently. Since cases are often provided free inside the box of saline, replace the case frequently. It is tempting, but never use tap water for storing or rinsing your contact lenses, as there are parasites and bacteria in even the cleanest water. The quickest dunk under the faucet with the contact lens on your finger is possibly dangerous.

When contact lenses start to get cloudy by the end of the day, they are telling you something. The protein building up on the contact lenses is good food for bacteria and those invaders will be eating away at your eye soon if you continue to wear them. When in doubt, change the contact lenses early if you need to. And don't ignore pain or redness! These symptoms are a sign of bad things to come. Extended wear contact lenses need to be changed to new ones as directed by your doctor. Daily contact lenses are lenses that are changed daily, minimizing the possibility of infection, but precautions of washing your hands prior to inserting or removing the lenses still need to be heeded.

Viruses and bacteria that cause pinkeye or conjunctivitis are spread from person to person and can be prevented by washing hands frequently, especially when exposed to anyone with a cold, flu-like virus, or pinkeye. I always emphasize the need for you constantly to wash your hands before you touch your eye. If you have allergies causing nasal and eye symptoms, this could make your eye susceptible to infection. Be sure to have these evaluated and treated by your doctor without delay.

Many older persons suffer from dry eye, and this can now be treated with prescription eye drops. Some cases of dry eye are simple to treat. Other cases result from conditions called sicca syndrome or the illness Sjogren's syndrome are treated by stronger eye drops. These two syndromes are caused by a lack of production of tears. Because these dry eye syndromes can lead to an inflamed, red eye, they can also lead to infections. Adequate treatment of the underlying condition by your eye doctor could prevent infections. Additionally, dry eye can develop after having LASIK procedures to correct vision; be sure to discuss your chance of this happening with your eye doctor if you are considering this procedure and have it evaluated if you are experiencing this side effect of LASIK.

Those who have had or are about to have cataract surgery need to be educated about this surgical procedure and its risk of infection. Infections are rare because the incisions are tiny and close up within minutes after surgery. However, the incision enters the eyeball such that if an infection does occur it can invade easily as mentioned above. LASIK and Radial keratotomy (RK), an uncommon procedure these days, involve cuts into the cornea that do not enter the eye. However, if an infection does develop in any of these surgeries, it can be very difficult to treat. Following any of these procedures follow the doctor's directions closely.

Cornea transplants have slightly larger incisions but newer techniques create even smaller openings and most now do not even enter the eyeball. Because there can be reactions to the implanted tissue, this complicates matters as the reaction can look similar to infection. The reaction can also put you at risk for infection because of the inflammation. The potential harm can be the same or worse than the other eye surgeries, but the risk is higher due to potential rejection of the donor cornea and the eye drops that the patients have to use. Again, follow the directions of your eye doctor closely after surgery.

There is no easy way to prevent these infections other than the above, but the key to protecting yourself and your eyes is getting to the eye doctor quickly if you have the beginnings of a possible infection. If you have allergies, it is important to treat the allergy symptoms appropriately because, if the allergic reactions in the eye get severe enough, they could turn into an infection. AND DON'T RUB YOUR EYES LIKE YOUR MOTHER SAID!!

Chapter 19

❧

Tuberculosis

Tuberculosis (TB) is the world's second most lethal infection in terms of total deaths (only behind malaria) and one of the more prevalent infections worldwide. According to the CDC and WHO, one third of the world's population is infected with TB. Worldwide 1.5 million people die of TB every year and, while it is declining in the US, in 2013, 9,582 cases of TB were diagnosed and there were approximately 500 deaths. Because of the slow growth of this bacterium, *Mycobacterium tuberculosis*, the growth cycle is unusual. The risks posed by TB are difficult to understand by both the general population and the medical community. One can live their whole life with a dormant TB bacteria in their lungs and never know it. If that bacteria breaks out of the walled off shell that the body creates for containment, it will create a contagious, possibly fatal disease.

All too often, in the United States, TB is not high on the list of possible diagnoses for any particular illness, thus delaying the diagnosis when it does cause infection. TB can cause disease in almost every body system, from the most common, the lungs, to the brain, intestines, bladder, kidneys, and bones. In foreign countries, such as India, because of its prevalence, TB is among the top on the list. Because of this, even with less advanced diagnostic technology, it is commonly considered and diagnosed earlier after presentation. Here in the US, it can be a real tragedy when the diagnosis is missed. I had a dear medical colleague who was born in India, and was a beloved primary care physician to many patients. She was hospitalized with tuberculous meningitis, but was not diagnosed soon enough to save her. While I was not on the case, I have to admit that even I would not have had the diagnosis on the tip of my tongue, even though she was foreign born. Had she been diagnosed earlier, she may have survived. This example illustrates the point that uncommon infections may only be considered later in a disease evaluation or undertreated due to lack of knowledge of the diagnosis and the treatment of this bacterium.

When a person with active TB infection breathes the bacteria out of their lungs, it is carried in the air for greater distances than the usual viral particles that travel by droplets in the air. With TB, this is called airborne transmission because the infectious fluid particles, called "droplet nuclei" are so small they can travel – actually float in the air - for several meters. This bacterium can then be inhaled into the lungs of a close contact, such as a family member or healthcare employee. Within days, the bacteria become walled off in the lungs by the recipient's immune system into what is called a granuloma. This microscopic cocoon either kills the bacteria or is tricked into allowing the TB bacteria to stay alive, albeit dormant. This is known as latent TB infection. From this point forward, for the rest of their life, this person has a 10% risk of this bacteria coming to life, breaking out of the granuloma, and causing active infection. About half of those who develop an active infection, will develop it within the first two years after breathing in the bacteria. The rest of the 10% will develop the infection later in life when they least expect it, as late as their nineties.

An average of 3.0 people per 100,000 population will be afflicted with active TB each year in the US. There are 9 states and Washington, DC that are above this rate, with Hawaii the highest at 8.2 per 100,000 population. The Marshall Islands have a case rate of 219 per 100,000. 70% of cases in the US are in foreign born individuals, with the vast majority of these having been in the US for greater than 5 years. Worldwide Swaziland has the highest rate with 1382 cases of active TB per 100,000 population with many countries in Central and South America, Africa, and Asia in the 100-200 cases per 100,000 population range. For example, India has a case rate of 177 per 100,000 population. To put this in perspective, in a majority of the underdeveloped countries of the world, if you lived in a town of 5,000 people there would be at least 5-10 people with active TB each year. In the US, the equivalent statistic would be in a town of 30,000 people there would be 1 person with active TB each year. To continue to decrease the rate of TB we need earlier detection. And with this early detection, we need more treatment of latent TB infection.

Purified protein derivative (PPD) testing has been around for 60 years. Proteins of the TB bacteria (not live bacteria) are prepared and injected into the dermal layer – the top layer – of skin on the forearm. If this person has been exposed to TB (latent TB infection), then a raised lesion will occur at the site of the injection. This does not mean the patient has a contagious, or active disease. More likely, the patient has TB bacteria walled off in the lungs in a granuloma (again, latent TB infection). The test is about 60-90% sensitive and 90% specific. In other words about 10-40% of the persons with active or latent disease will have a negative test. And about 10% of those with no TB (latent or active) will have a positive test.

There is an easier, better test that is gaining popularity. The Interferon Gamma Release Assay or IGRA (there are two brands: Quantiferon Gold and T-Spot) is a blood test that can also detect exposure to TB. It is more sensitive and more specific than the PPD. This means less false positive (a positive test in a patient who is not infected with TB infection) and less false negative (a negative test in someone with TB infection) tests. With the ease of a blood test, patients are more likely to have the test performed if they need it. The PPD has to be injected into the top layer of the skin, causing people with fears of needles to not be tested, and it has to be evaluated by a nurse or doctor 48 to 72 hours later, which can cause difficulty arranging appointments to evaluate the test and patient compliance with recommendations. My ability to test my HIV patients for exposure to TB has increased several-fold using IGRA testing.

There are two groups of people who need regular PPD or IGRA testing - persons who are more likely to be exposed to people with active TB such as close contacts of a case of active TB, health care workers, immigrants from countries with high rates of TB, and residents and employees of correctional facilities and homeless shelters; and people who are more likely to be stricken with active TB if they do become exposed, such as HIV positive individuals, injection drug users, and patients with rheumatoid arthritis or Crohn's disease treated with certain medications, diabetes mellitus, silicosis, chronic kidney disease, a history of surgical gastrectomy or a history of solid organ transplants. All of these individuals should have periodic PPD or IGRA testing periodically as often as yearly.

HIV patients carry a 10% risk per year of getting an active infection if they have a positive PPD without having treatment. Consequently, HIV patients should have a PPD or Interferon Gamma Release Assay (IGRA) yearly. HIV patients also carry a greater risk of more severe forms of TB. If health care providers can catch the exposure early in these patients, then we can treat with antibiotics to prevent active TB.

Now with this detection of more individuals earlier after the breathing in of bacteria into their lungs (latent TB infection), we need further treatment. In general, the CDC recommends treatment of all individuals with a positive PPD or IGRA unless we can document adequate treatment in the past. There are a few treatment options, but the usual is 9 months of a combination of Isoniazid (INH) and Vitamin B6 (pyridoxine) to prevent the neuropathy symptoms of INH. At least monthly monitoring of liver blood tests should accompany the treatment. This treatment lowers the risk of progressing from latent to active TB by over 80%. There is a safer, simpler treatment available that has a duration of only 2 months if the patient qualifies, but must be closely monitored for adherence.

One of the main reasons for the high rate of tuberculosis in foreign countries is the lack of PPD testing and the lack of adequate health care resources to treat these individuals. In many countries, the cost of the INH would be borne by the individual who is making pennies per day in manual labor. Unless they obtain a medication for free, they are not likely to be able to afford it. In addition, in foreign countries there is an even larger belief in homeopathic medicine than in the US, and these patients are distrustful of the medical establishment. The same can also be now said for the US. In addition, there is a woeful lack of education of the frontline primary care physicians as to the need for this treatment especially in those more urban and lower socioeconomic areas of New York City and Washington, DC and our island commonwealths.

For a few years I had the pleasure of working on a Caribbean island where the risk of tuberculosis was almost as high as Washington, DC and New York City, but not as high as some foreign countries. In the local government hospital and in the health department clinic, I encountered multiple persons diagnosed with active tuberculosis. Despite this high risk of contracting tuberculosis, I had a fireman and a nurse refuse to be treated for latent tuberculosis infection. I had a physician in the community tell both of these patients that treatment was not necessary. The lack of evaluation and treatment knowledge among health care professionals is commonplace in foreign countries, but is also not unheard of in the mainland US. For this and other reasons related to a high rate of HIV infections, the Caribbean Islands as well as other areas with an ill-informed population will continue to have a high rate of active, contagious TB.

Protecting yourself from TB exposure would be difficult, given the airborne spread of this bacteria. More significant TB exposure usually would come from crowded situations, such as in prison, homeless shelters, and group housing. If you are travelling to foreign countries, especially as part of medical missions, be aware of this increased risk of exposure. Any mention of symptoms of cough, bloody phlegm, night sweats, or weight loss should prompt you to protect yourself by using a mask. The type of mask to use is called N95 – it filters at least 95% of small particles from the air. If you have difficulty breathing through the mask, there are special masks with valves that are still N95 certified. See the chapter on protective equipment for more information.

Once you have been diagnosed with a positive PPD or IGRA, you will almost always have a positive test from that day forward. Indeed, after an initial reaction to the PPD, you could get a worse reaction on your next PPD than the initial positive result. Therefore, instead of the PPD or IGRA you should have a baseline and an annual chest X-ray after you have been treated for the latent TB infection.

I have seen many patients come in with active TB within a few years after a negative PPD, so be vigilant about your risk and continue to get tested if you are at risk. The worst case I have seen was a patient who was homeless and had been seen at 2 local hospitals with a diagnosis of bronchitis, with symptoms of weight loss, bloody cough, and night sweats (classic for active tuberculosis). He told us that several years prior, as a younger man, he had a negative PPD. He was admitted a month later at our hospital with miliary tuberculosis, which means it had actively spread throughout the body. This person survived but not without a lengthy hospital stay and at high cost to society.

To protect yourself from becoming actively infected with TB, if you are part of a high-risk group mentioned above, get tested for latent TB as frequently as yearly, preferably with the IGRA. And if positive, suggest to your physician that you would like to be treated, or refer yourself to a pulmonologist (lung doctor), infectious disease physician, or the county health department physician. The CDC recommends that almost everyone be treated if their PPD or IGRA test is positive, even those who have had a vaccine for TB in the past. Follow their directions, but be mindful about the lack of education out there. Often university medical clinics are more aware of current guidelines. They are more likely to have experience treating indigent and foreign-born patients and therefore have experience with treating positive TB tests.

Check out the CDC's website to educate yourself further:

http://www.cdc.gov/tb/topic/treatment/

http://www.cdc.gov/tb/topic/treatment/ltbi.htm.

Chapter 20

∾

Hepatitis Viruses

Hepatitis has become a household word in many areas of the world as millions if not billions of people have become infected with one of the hepatitis viruses. There are five main hepatitis viruses that infect humans. Hepatitis A and E are viruses that are spread by the fecal-oral route, meaning that one can contract these viruses by close contact with someone with the virus or by ingestion of food or other contaminated products. Hepatitis B, C, and D are spread parenterally, meaning it requires blood-to-blood or other body fluid contact to transmit the virus from one person to another. Hepatitis B and D can be spread sexually. There have been reports of Hepatitis C being spread sexually but sexual transmission is felt to be less common.

In general, Hepatitis A causes an illness with mild liver damage that resolves within several weeks. However one in a 1000 patients who contract Hepatitis A could develop fulminant hepatitis causing the quick onset of liver failure causing death unless a liver transplant can be performed. There are dozens of reports of outbreaks yearly of Hepatitis A from food service workers, fresh fruits and vegetables, and from children at daycare centers. Once an individual recovers from an infection, he or she will be immune from reacquiring the disease. It is so common in the United States that by 30 years of age, 30% of people in the United States will have evidence of past infection. In other countries it is even more common due to less than adequate hygiene and farming practices.

Similar to healthcare workers, fast food restaurant employees have a dismal track record when it comes to hand washing compliance. Handling of your food by a person with an illness with Hepatitis A (or E) prior to serving it to you is a common way for you to contract this illness. Imagine an employee at your favorite restaurant who has what seems to him just a minor stomach bug. He still comes to work because he needs to earn his weekly paycheck or he is afraid of being fired. He could be in charge of salads or the grill, or he could be the dishwasher. In any case, if he touches your plate or food with unclean hands, the virus could be lurking waiting for you to ingest it. Often persons with Hepatitis A have a subclinical illness, which means they do not have any symptoms at all. In addition, people with Hepatitis A and other viruses could shed viruses for a day or so before symptoms start and for days after symptoms resolve. That salad chef that made your salad may not even know he is sick.

Even worse at hand washing are small children, especially at daycares and schools. Children are notorious for touching feces or bathroom surfaces, not washing their hands, then touching other small children. If one child has Hepatitis A, it will not be difficult to spread it to other children, or adults for that matter. In rural and migrant communities children are in contact with farm animals and other children setting up a recipe for the spread of this virus. In addition, in farms in the United States and elsewhere, it is possible that fresh produce can come in contact with human waste from an overcrowded community or with animal waste or manure that could contain Hepatitis A or E. Often in third world countries, livestock and their excrement are near the fields that your blueberries are planted in. Human waste could be near the fields, or worse yet, used as fertilizer for the strawberries that reach your grocery store shelf.

Most cases of Hepatitis A will never enter my hospital or clinic, because the illness is subclinical or not noticeable enough to warrant a doctor visit. However, the cases I do see are often the worst cases, the ones that ultimately require a liver transplant. Take, for example, the older gentleman in Florida who ate coleslaw, potato salad, and fried chicken at a church picnic and 5 days later had severe liver damage and quickly deteriorating condition. This patient underwent a liver transplant and after a few months in the hospital, lived to tell the tale of how a plate of coleslaw almost killed him.

Hepatitis E is rare in the United States but is found commonly in Mexico, Cuba, Africa, and South Asia. Similar to Hepatitis A, it causes a self-limited illness, but pregnant women are at risk for fulminant disease. In the United States, Hepatitis E causes a few outbreaks along the Texas or California border, or from produce imported from Mexico. Rarely, in patients whose immune systems are suppressed due to transplants, a chronic illness can occur.

You can help protect yourself from Hepatitis A and E with some simple steps. First, wash all of your fresh fruits and vegetables with a vegetable wash. You can create your own wash with bleach that is diluted. Rinse off with tap water afterward. If you travel to a foreign country, do not eat fresh vegetable or fruits unless they are peeled. That especially includes fresh salads. See the travel section of this book for more specific recommendations. Second, utilize alcohol hand sanitizer frequently, especially if you come in contact with children. Third, if you travel outside the United States or if you are in the healthcare or childcare industry, there is a highly recommended vaccine that protects one from Hepatitis A, that is given in two doses 6 months apart. It confers lifelong immunity in greater than 90% of people who take it. Hepatitis E does not have a protective vaccine, therefore only the other precautions apply.

Hepatitis B, C, and D are spread parenterally, meaning by body fluid or blood exposure. Since the 1960s there has been a continuous spread of these viruses among IV drug users who share needles. But that is not the only way drug users can spread these viruses. Hepatitis C has been spread via multiple avenues to millions of Americans. Cocaine straws and dollar bills, when shared among the often-bleeding noses of cocaine users, can spread all three viruses. Hepatitis B, D, and less commonly possibly Hepatitis C can be spread sexually. While not as common as it once was, transmission from a contaminated tattoo needle or ink can occur. Hepatitis B can be transmitted through close household contact with a person with acute or chronic Hepatitis B, especially when razors or toothbrushes are shared. There are a multitude of persons who become infected with no known contact to an individual with Hepatitis B or C. It is these infections that are scary.

Hepatitis B is extremely common in Asia. While not as common in the US, there are 700,000 people chronically infected with Hepatitis B with 20,000 new infections yearly. Globally, there are more than 350 million persons with chronic Hepatitis B and more than 4 million acute cases yearly with 1 million deaths each year attributable to Hepatitis B. This rivals tuberculosis and malaria for the most prolific killers of the human race presently, which have 1.5 million and 500,000 deaths per year, respectively.

I have seen a multitude of patients who have had acute and chronic Hepatitis B, from the retired physician to the mother of three, to the drug using young adult. Hepatitis B is becoming less common due to the common practice of vaccinating babies against this disease. It is almost unheard of to not receive Hepatitis B at birth; however, it requires follow-up at the pediatrician to complete the series. The second and third doses need to be given in the first 15 months of life. It is unfortunate when I see an 18 year old who presents with acute fulminant Hepatitis B, when it could have been prevented during infancy. One patient in particular comes to mind because he now has to be on lifelong treatment for it.

There are more than 3.2 million persons in the United States chronically infected with Hepatitis C, representing 1 in every 100 persons. Only 1.6 million persons with Hepatitis C have been diagnosed and only 170,000 have been successfully treated. Newer, better medications are cutting down on the gap of people not treated. However, what is clearly needed is more testing. If the recommendations of the USPTF (United States Prevention Task Force) are heeded, which are to test all persons born between 1945 and 1965 and all persons with risk factors, there would be an additional 1.3 million persons diagnosed. If more patients were treated, this would prevent tens of thousands of new infections and thousands of cases of liver failure.

Similar to Hepatitis B, the patients I have had with Hepatitis C come from all walks of life, including celebrities, young mothers, doctors, attorneys, and current and former drug users. In the US, though, it is more common than Hepatitis B; we all know many people with Hepatitis C whether we or they are aware of it or not. In the 1990s and 2000s we did not have the best track record for treatment, as only 40% or less of the patients treated were able to eradicate the virus. We now have medications that have a 90% or greater success rate. Unfortunately this is too late for the thousands who have died prior to the advent of these medications.

Hepatitis D is essentially the same as Hepatitis B because it is a mutated hepatitis virus that requires chronic infection with Hepatitis B to lend it a required factor for growth. It is relatively rare and difficult to diagnose due to lack of consideration by doctors to evaluate for it. Because it requires Hepatitis B to survive, prevention of Hepatitis B is the key to protecting yourself from this virus.

The best method to protect yourself from these 3 viruses (B, C, and D) is to avoid exposure to blood and body fluids of other persons. Avoid sharing of needles and drug paraphernalia such as cocaine straws and dollar bills. It is not only the needles and straws but sharing any item of drug use including the drug itself, which could become contaminated. Tattoo parlors have been an important source of transmission of these viruses in the past, but strict regulation has made this less likely. Unfortunately, it still occurs, therefore you should only use the services of reputable tattoo artists. Monitor the needle and ink, both of which should be unsealed in front of you. The artist should also be wearing gloves.

Use of condoms may be effective at preventing Hepatitis B, but the following data from needle sticks may suggest that you should not rely only on condoms to prevent sexual acquisition of Hepatitis B. Hepatitis B is 10 times more transmissible than Hepatitis C and 100 times more transmissible than HIV via needle sticks. The same ratio may not be true for sexual transmission but it can give you an idea about how easy it is to catch Hepatitis B.

If you engage in risky behavior (anyone who has been or will be sexually active with more than one partner, ever) or if a family member or close contact (such as a roommate) has chronic Hepatitis B, you can protect yourself with a vaccination series. The entire series should be given (either 3 shots alone or 2 if given in a combination shot with Hepatitis A) in order to protect yourself. If a family member has acute (new infection with) Hepatitis B, there is an immune globulin (a shot with protective antibodies from donated blood or plasma) that can be used to protect you from infection. It is expensive and not for everyone. There is no vaccination for Hepatitis C or D currently.

Those in certain fields such as healthcare, police, firemen and corrections workers are required to have the three shot series for Hepatitis B. Missionaries and long term travelers to West Africa, and possibly other areas of Africa and Southeast Asia should also be vaccinated because as much as 1 in every 10 people in these countries is infected. Also, patients with liver disease and those on dialysis should also receive the vaccine. It has a greater than 90% chance of being protective and a simple blood test can determine if you are indeed protected. The series is only needed once during your lifetime. As mentioned before, most babies in the US are given the initial vaccine but then require two more shots from their pediatrician. Presumably they should have lifelong protection.

New Hepatitis C vaccine research shows some promise but we are still a long way from this elusive goal of preventing virus acquisition. For now, we need to be vigilant and the main goal now is to increase the number of patients diagnosed and treated to prevent new infections. Again, protect yourself with proven prevention.

For More Information:

http://www.cdc.gov/vaccines/vpd-vac/hepb/

http://europepmc.org/articles/pmc3285467

http://www.ncbi.nlm.nih.gov/pmc/articles/PMC4586034/

Holmberg SD, et al. NEJM, 2013, 368(20):1859-61.

http://annals.org/article.aspx?articleid=723191

Chapter 21

~

Shingles

You may not remember it well, but your parents have vivid memories of when you had multiple lesions of chickenpox all over your body when you were young. Your body's immune system remembers it well, too, but with every year its memory is fading. Shingles is caused by the chickenpox virus (also called varicella-zoster virus or VZV) and after your initial infection with chickenpox, it stays dormant in your body for the rest of your life in clusters of nerve cell bodies called "ganglia" that line each side of your spine from the base of your skull to the bottom of your spine. Your immune system prevents it from coming out into a noticeable infection. However, your immune system's memory is somewhat limited by age just like our brain's memory wanes as we get older. It starts to forget about all of the viruses we contracted when we were a child and young adult. Because there are many viruses that continue to survive in small numbers in our body, if the memory fades, then some of these viruses could reactivate or return to cause a mild infection. Since the immune memory is still present to some degree, the reactivation of infection is almost always mild, unless there are other factors present, such as chemotherapy or other immune suppressing medications. Examples of these viruses include the herpes viruses, Epstein Barr Virus (mono) and varicella-zoster virus. It is controversial for some viruses as to whether any reactivation occurs or whether it is clinically significant, but VZV is well documented.

Anyone who has ever had shingles may take exception to the term mild in the previous paragraph, as the pain associated with this disease may be excruciating and debilitating. As described above, VZV survives in the dorsal root ganglia (a collection of nerve cells) near the spinal cord in the sensory nerve cells. If VZV becomes reactivated in older age, it will travel down the nerve to its endings in the skin and causes blistering lesions on the skin only in the section that is innervated by that nerve or bundle of nerves. This is called a dermatome and it is often linear, wrapping around one side of the body and never crossing the midline. The nerve that is involved sends signals that it is damaged to the brain and the brain interprets these signals as burning, stabbing, aching, or gnawing types of pain.

The lesions often last about a week to 10 days, but the pain can persist for weeks. In some cases the pain persists for months or years and is called post-herpetic neuralgia - PHN (VZV is part of the herpes family of viruses (but not sexually transmitted) hence the term herpetic). There are medications that can help treat these symptoms but I will not discuss these here. The debilitating nature of the pain has prompted the use of antiviral medications such as acyclovir, valacyclovir, and famciclovir to treat shingles if it erupts. Studies have shown that early use of valacyclovir during an episode of shingles (preferably within the first 72 hours of an outbreak) will prevent or lessen the neuralgia (pain) that will result.

There are very limited numbers of persons who have had multiple episodes of shingles. These persons may benefit from taking one of the medications above in a low dose daily to prevent recurrence of shingles. In addition, there are other diagnoses that mimic shingles such as Herpes Simplex or dermatitis herpetiformis and other various vasculitis (or auto-immune) lesions. If you have recurrent outbreaks, it could be one of these conditions or another cause of a rash such as an allergy. Have your doctor look at the lesions or biopsy them. There are possible treatments you could take to prevent these.

However, there is a way you can protect yourself from shingles occurring in the first place by jarring your immune system's memory using almost the same vaccine that has previously been given to children to prevent chicken pox. It is a live vaccine (the virus is alive but weakened) and therefore is not available for certain immunocompromised patients. The FDA has approved it for use in persons 60 years of age and older. The shingles vaccine decreases the incidence of shingles by 64% in ages 60-69 and by 38% in those aged 70-79. The vaccine wanes in effectiveness 5 years after it is given but there is no recommendation to receive repeat dosing after 5 years. There is a newer vaccine in development that so far has a 97% reduction in episodes of shingles.

If you have what you suspect is shingles, do not wait. Protect yourself from the possible weeks of pain that may ensue. See your doctor right away and ask if acyclovir, valacyclovir, or famciclovir would prevent postherpetic neuralgia. Acyclovir does not absorb well through the stomach, so you may be better off taking valacyclovir or famciclovir if you can afford it. Steroids or prednisone usually is only reserved for patients who have extensive shingles involving a large area of skin (multiple dermatomes). If your shingles episode is close to your eye or involves the tip of your nose or your ear, you may be at risk for rare complications that could affect your vision or your hearing. Seek medical care from a specialist in ophthalmology, or ear nose and throat (ENT), or Infectious Diseases.

If you have what looks like a bacterial infection called cellulitis of the face, instead it could be shingles. At some point in the infection, it should manifest the more typical lesions (small blister like lesion) only on one side of the face. Sometimes shingles can become secondarily infected by bacteria, thus having both shingles and cellulitis. These dual infections can be worrisome.

Again, protect yourself from shingles using the vaccine and treatment with antiviral medications to prevent the subsequent pain. Avoiding the burning pain that many experience is well worth it.

For more information:

http://www.cdc.gov/vaccines/vpd-vac/shingles/hcp-vax-recs.html#effectiveness

http://www.nejm.org/doi/full/10.1056/NEJMoa1501184

Chapter 22

~

Tetanus, Diphtheria, and Pertussis

Tetanus, diphtheria, and pertussis are as different as the day is old. However, they have been connected for the last 40 years in millions of small vials aimed at preventing these often deadly diseases. Each of these bacteria raises their ugly heads to infect patients who have not been vaccinated adequately. I see it all too often. Unfortunately insurance companies don't cover these vaccinations unless you have cut yourself and present to the emergency room.

Just last year I treated two patients for tetanus, one of which was a 20 something year old patient who had a small impalement by a nail and one week later he was intubated and fighting for his life in the intensive care unit, after contracting wound tetanus, or lockjaw. He spent 6 months in the hospital, mostly in intensive care because he could not breathe on his own, and probably spent the next 6 months regaining the strength he had lost. *Clostridium tetani*, the bacterial causative agent, is so common in soil and on impaling objects such as nails that ER physicians routinely give tetanus vaccines for any laceration.

Because of this proactive treatment in the ER, tetanus is extremely rare in the US. However what happens to all of those persons who have not been vaccinated and do not seek treatment after their cut? Approximately 20 to 30 cases are reported every year in the US and this continues to decline. The fatality rate is 13% overall but is over 30% in those over 65 which is the most common age group to be stricken by tetanus. This illness is not spread from person to person, your duty to be vaccinated is more to protect yourself if you have a laceration or puncture wound.

One may argue, why be so paranoid about tetanus when there are only 20 cases per year. However, as recently as 1995 there were 60 cases, in the 1970's there were approximately 100 cases per year, and in the 1950's about 500 cases occurred annually. So you can see, the steady rate of decline occurred in the last 100 years, owing primarily to vaccines, although the urbanization of our population may have had a part also.

Diphtheria is even more rare, but occurs mainly in non-immunized persons, especially immigrants. Eastern European and Russian immigrants commonly are victims of this malady in the US because they have not had adequate immunizations. This bacterium (*Clostridium diphtheriae*) causes severe pharyngitis and can spread to the rest of the body very quickly. The illness often requires intubation with sepsis and severe clotting abnormalities are the norm. Diphtheria is spread by contact with secretions or by inhalation of tiny droplets of an infected patient. Herd immunity can protect an entire population if enough people are vaccinated. I will explain herd immunity later in this chapter.

While only a handful of cases of diphtheria have occurred in the US in the last decade, there are thousands of cases annually in the world. In the 1920's vaccinations became available and the illness has decreased from that time frame. In 1921 there were 200,000 cases and 15,000 deaths. In the US, the illness has become extremely rare, but may increase as the anti-vaccine movements may quickly change our herd immunity and undo decades of protection from this deadly disease. It takes 85% of the population to be vaccinated to prevent diphtheria outbreaks. If less than this amount of the population is vaccinated, then it is more likely to expect sporadic infections. There are small but growing areas of the US that are dipping below the 85%. Some are as low as 50 to 60% and soon this will create an untenable situation.

Unlike the previous two bacteria, *Bordetella pertussis*, which causes pertussis or "whooping cough", is becoming more common, also due to loss of protective immunity from childhood vaccinations. Even after vaccination, it appears the immunity from these primary series vaccinations given in childhood or from boosters often given in young adulthood may only be protective for less than twenty years. Because of this, whooping cough is a disease that is now seen in middle age quite routinely usually by 40 years of age. Pertussis is very contagious; the average person who contracts pertussis passes it on to 6 other persons. The herd immunity required to prevent pertussis is 92%. This means that 92% of the population must be effectively vaccinated to prevent the spread of the bacteria among the population.

Physicians often diagnose whooping cough based on symptoms of a cough that is severe enough to cause a barking noise and often results in vomiting. However, in middle age, the symptoms can often be indistinguishable from the common cold or bronchitis – adults do not "whoop". It is diagnosed on either sputum or a swab or other sample of nasal secretions that detect the DNA of pertussis. I have had patients that were incorrectly diagnosed as a viral infection, admitted to the hospital and this simple swab has resulted in them being accurately diagnosed and treated. The bacterium is very easy to treat but often causes symptoms even after eradication of the bacteria, resulting in a prolonged illness of coughing fits that lasts weeks after treatment. Patients often ask for and receive a second round of antibiotics, even though the additional antibiotics are usually unnecessary.

Take one of my patients who was treated for a bronchitis with antibiotics that would effectively treat pertussis was admitted due to her having HIV and asthma. Testing confirmed she had pertussis. She was treated with another round of antibiotics in the hospital and finally after two more weeks she had resolution of her symptoms. She probably would have improved over that two weeks regardless of whether she had that second round of antibiotics. More importantly, had she been properly vaccinated she would have been protected and would not have become ill in the first place.

Childhood vaccines include all three of the bacteria, and then historically included only tetanus and diphtheria in teenage years. In adulthood, in previous years the only booster given was for tetanus and diphtheria. So if you go to the emergency room after a cut or to the doctor's office to update your vaccinations you were only protected from tetanus and diphtheria but not pertussis. However, now, there is a combination of all three with an acellular pertussis component (called Tdap) that can be given to adults. It is more expensive though, and therefore adoption by emergency rooms and insurance companies has been slow. This is likely why my patient above, who had Medicare that does not cover Tdap, did not choose to be vaccinated.

To protect yourself from these three bacteria, it is important to vaccinate your children and to maintain a Tdap vaccination at least every 10 years; it is recommended with every pregnancy no matter the time frame. If you sustain a laceration that is dirty, in other words, with anything that is not sterile, if you have not had a tetanus booster within 5 years, you should receive a booster in the form of Tdap. A quick trip to the walk-in clinic or emergency room and you will be protecting yourself for years to come and not just from tetanus but also diphtheria and pertussis. Ask to make sure you are receiving Tdap and not just Td, which does not cover pertussis. Cleaning a wound will help reduce the risk, but the spores often remain in the wound after washing and are not killed by soaps.

Herd immunity is the concept of the protection of all persons in a community by immunizing enough persons in the community (either naturally by past infections or artificially through vaccinations) so that very few infections occur. Depending on the virus or bacteria, there are a certain percentage of individuals that need to be vaccinated to provide herd immunity. Measles, Mumps, Rubella, and Polio all have a requirement also around 85% vaccination rate to prevent infections. H1N1 influenza, which is not as contagious, requires only a 40% vaccination rate to prevent infections in the community. Currently in 2014, in the US 93% of children have had adequate polio vaccination and 91% have had adequate MMR (Measles, mumps and rubella), and about 88% of teens have had a Tdap vaccine. Only about 3% of adults had had a Tdap in the past two years in 2007. Obviously these numbers vary by state and can be lower than the herd immunity requirement in some states and are better in states with better healthcare (or fewer anti-vaxxers). If you look worldwide the rates are very low but improving because of WHO efforts. In Africa, 77% had adequate polio and DTP coverage, but certain countries in Africa are at 50%, which seems outstanding compared to where we once were. Haiti has finally, in 2014, obtained an 85% rubella vaccination rate and an 85%

polio rate. These countries are, encouragingly, headed in the opposite direction as the US. You can search for you own state's rates. Some links below can help.

Remember, even though the rates of diphtheria and tetanus in the US are low, it is because of these vaccines that this is the case. And pertussis or whooping cough is more common recently because of increasing recognition of these infections and their potentially fatal outcome in the elderly. Protect yourself by becoming educated about these infections and get vaccinated. In addition, be aware of your risks when you are exposed such as when you get a cut from a dirty object.

More information:

Concepts of herd protection and immunity. Procedia in Vaccinology 2010, Vol.2(2):134–139. Global Vaccine Research Forum, Bamako, Mali, 6-9 December 2009. **http://www.sciencedirect.com/science/article/pii/S1877282X10000299**

http://www.cdc.gov/vaccines/imz-managers/coverage/imz-coverage.html

http://www.who.int/immunization/monitoring_surveillance/data/en/

Chapter 23

~

Ebola

In 2014, there were 5 cases of Ebola in the United States, 3 persons who returned from Africa with the disease, and 2 cases that were transmitted from one of those persons to healthcare providers in the US. The press deemed that to be a failure of the CDC and proclaimed that there was going to be an outbreak in the US. Luckily for us (and owing nothing to luck, but everything to the CDC and state health departments), this did not occur. In addition, more than 11,000 people died mostly in 3 countries in Africa during almost 3 years of an outbreak that to this day in March 2016 still threatens to re-emerge.

Since it was first discovered in 1976, Ebola and other hemorrhagic viruses (including Marburg), have caused a devastating and often fatal illness that has been centered on Central and West Africa. Ebola can be found in fruit bats (without harming them as far as we know) in these areas. From the bats, which eat fruit in the trees, it is spread to other animals that eat half-eaten fruit or the bats themselves. Likely it is spread from these animals and bats to primates. Humans may eat or come in contact with these wild animals, thus contracting the virus themselves.

From there it can be spread from close contact with infectious fluids of patients with the disease. It is widely thought that Ebola virus cannot be spread by infected persons unless they have disease symptoms. It can be present in the bodily fluids of deceased persons. It also has been found in some bodily fluids (such as semen) of persons who have been sick from Ebola and have subsequently recovered. The virus could be present in semen for a year or more after recovery, but we are not sure if it can be spread from this reservoir. For many reasons, we have an extreme difficulty containing the epidemics in Africa. There is a lot of distrust in the medical providers working to prevent spread of the virus in Africa. Keeping populations isolated from others has proven difficult. It is also difficult to change the customs and traditions regarding burial and funeral processions which often involve touching or carrying the dead bodies.

From 1976 to 2016 there were 35 different outbreaks of this virus. All of them pale in comparison to the outbreak in West Africa in 2014 and 2015. Most of the outbreaks have been in Central Africa in Uganda and the Democratic Republic of Congo, which, including the rest of West Africa is the territory of the African fruit bat. There have also been a few cases in the Philippines possibly related to pigs. During a few outbreaks and especially during the outbreak of 2014, there have been cases of Ebola in health care workers and missionaries that have been involved in the care of patients with the disease.

What has not occurred has been a case of Ebola imported to the US in an Ebola-free individual without known exposure to the illness. All infected persons from the US have been in workers known to be working with ill persons. This is not to say that it could not occur in a casual vacationing traveler, but it would be unusual. The worst-case scenario would be a full outbreak in the US. Without a reservoir of fruit bats, the outbreak would not sustain itself for long with the modern public health infrastructure. One could imagine a few hundred cases maximum unless people refused to be tested or isolated. Similar to the movie "Outbreak", the virus would have to become airborne to spread more widely.

What is unclear is whether there is any possibility of spread of the disease to others from an individual who has already recovered from the virus but harbors the virus inside his body. If the virus indeed is harbored in some bodily fluids, can these bodily fluids spread the virus to close contacts? Theoretically this could happen and there are theories that some of the extra

The main method of protection would be to be aware of your surroundings and individuals you come into contact with while travelling or working in Central and West Africa. If you are a healthcare worker or missionary, most aid agencies in Central or West Africa are fully aware of the precautions you should take. In the situation of an outbreak, and you are not a healthcare or other worker in direct contact with sick patients, common ear loop masks and gloves should suffice, as the spread would be by droplet or contact of mucous membranes by bodily fluids. N95 masks can help prevent droplet and airborne spread. t this time, Ebola does not seem to be spread by the airborne route. In general however, most persons would be wise to use N95 masks as a precaution. However, the healthcare workers who became ill in the most recent outbreak, had taken precautions and they still contracted the disease, so the following prevention is recommended.

If you are in Africa (or anywhere else) caring for sick patients with one of these viruses, a far stricter regimen of protective garments will be necessary. Persons infected with Ebola also have vomiting, diarrhea, and bleeding from multiple orifices. Hence, double or triple gloves and gowns and fluid shields should be used if in direct care of a family member. Care should be taken to dispose of anything that is exposed to bodily fluids of the infected person. The health department likely will handle disposal of any linens, sheets, and clothes worn by the individual. Do not touch any of these items; if you must touch them, do so only with the triple gowns and gloves in place. Do not share any utensil or personal care item with the infected person. Careful measurement of temperatures of individuals exposed to infected patients to determine when to isolate them is essential. It seems like common sense, but isolating oneself and notifying public health officials with the first onset of signs of illness is essential.

Hospitals have policies of using either full body suits with self-contained respirators, triple gowning, and triple gloving along with masks and shields. They utilize a buddy system where there is supervised donning (putting on) and doffing (taking off) the equipment. At all times a careful order and method is used that will decrease the possibility of touching the skin to any material that was exposed to the patient. They use negative pressure rooms but this is not theoretically required.

If you use some element of this careful detail to avoid exposure, it may help you protect yourself. If you have a family member in your household who has contracted a hemorrhagic fever virus, you can perform some of the same triple gowning and gloving to prevent exposure. However, as with the 2 nurses in the US who became infected, even some of these measures were not enough. Be aware of the possible transmission of the virus from one of the following countries to the US: Sierra Leone, Uganda, Congo, Democratic Republic of Congo, Guinea, Liberia, Gabon, South Sudan, Sudan, Cote d'Ivoire, and the Philippines. Countries nearby that have serologic evidence of infection include Senegal, Mali, and Nigeria, Chad, Cameroon, Central African Republic, and Madagascar. (CDC, 2014; WHO, 2009 maps)

Experimental treatments using the serum of those who have previously recovered from Ebola have been attempted but are not accepted treatments. In addition, a new medication, ZMapp, is an antibody against Ebola that was used in two individuals in the 2014 outbreak. The two individuals were doing poorly and it was thought that they were not going to survive. However, after the administration of the experimental drug, they recovered. It is unknown whether it would be successful on a wider scale, but there are some encouraging results so far with a small improvement in mortality in one study. Further studies will be needed to elucidate the success of this medication.

In general the treatment is supportive with fluids and blood products that replace lost blood, platelets, and clotting factors. Survival depends on being in a facility equipped to handle the use of blood products and modern hemodynamic (blood pressure) support. This likely explains the high survival rate of persons extricated to the US. If you or a loved one contracts Ebola in a foreign country, evacuation to the US may offer the best survival. If you remain in country, pay close attention to the availability of blood products. If necessary, you can ask for direct donation of blood products from a relative, but keep a close eye on the donated blood and how it is handled and make sure it does not get stolen.

There are vaccines being worked on now to prevent illness in primates and humans. One such trial is underway in Sierra Leone. However, there will likely continue to be a reservoir of virus in the wild unless the virus can be eradicated from the fruit bats. As of January 2016, all 3 countries in Africa have been declared free of Ebola since it has been more than

42 days in each of the countries since the last known case.   New information has a few isolated cases occurring in 2016.

In the unlikely case of a global outbreak of Ebola or other hemorrhagic virus you have the knowledge to overcome it, you just need to be prepared with the tools going forward.   Don't rely on the media, become educated by more informed sources such as the CDC and WHO.   Protect yourself and your family the best you can.

More information:

https://www.cdc.gov/vhf/ebola/

Chapter 24

~

Personal Protective Equipment

The tools you will need to protect yourself from the multitude of lurking dangers that await you every second of every day depend on the relative risk and the particular bug you want to avoid. The relative risk stems from the likelihood that you will be exposed. It doesn't make sense to wear a mask unless there is an illness in the community and you will come into close proximity to this virus or bacteria or your condition warrants protection from routine viruses. Each bacteria or virus has a certain ability to travel through the air and also an ability to survive on either wet or dry surfaces. Their ability to travel through the air depends on the particle size. For pathogens that survive on surfaces or in liquids, the likelihood of exposure and the amount of splashing that may occur will be important. The right type of personal protective equipment (PPE) makes all the difference.

The most commonly used PPE includes head covers, masks, gowns, gloves, eyewear, and footwear. Your use of a combination of these products could protect you from the host of invaders that you cannot see or predict. It is useful to know the rationale for your need for this equipment and the capabilities of the equipment before you purchase it. I have seen many patients - even nurses and doctors - using equipment in the wrong situations, which is like wearing a catcher's mask to play basketball.

Every product of protective equipment has testing that is performed to determine how it resists fluid penetration, how breathable the material is, how efficient it is at preventing bacteria or viruses from penetrating, latex content and flammability. This information is submitted to the FDA to become approved, but there are varying degrees of protection. For example, there are simple paper masks that do not filter much and even 2-ply masks usually do not prevent fluid from penetrating. Even relatively large particles or bacteria/viruses can still penetrate some of these masks. I will start from the top with head covers, then eyewear and masks, and finally, body and foot coverings.

The function of head covers is not only to prevent splashing of fluid onto the head area, but also to prevent the hair of caregivers from contaminating a field in the hospital. Hairnet head covers have very little fluid resistance. Simple surgical head covers that cover only the hair and cover some of the ear are usually fluid resistant to splashing liquids. There are different weights of fabric utilized in the construction. There are head covers that extend all the way down to the neck with an opening for the eye and mouth area. This is meant for strict biohazard control and the fluid resistance is of the highest degree. It is often used with a respirator.

Protective eyewear can be stand-alone or can be combined as a face shield in a face shield mask or with a respirator. Goggles provide the best stand-alone protection from splashing in the eyes and safety glasses are also somewhat protective against splashing. The issue with any of these devices is whether splashes can get around the outside of the goggles to the eyes. These should be accredited by NIOSH, the National Institute for Occupational Safety and Health. They should resist breakage - this information should be provided on the product label. Respirators are also approved by NIOSH.

Masks are the most complex piece of equipment since there are multiple varieties and multiple specifications. In general, the FDA must approve the distribution of masks and companies that make the masks can either have no claims of protection or certain claims of protection can be made. Fluid resistance can be claimed if at least 29 of 32 masks tested resists penetration through the mask by a small amount of synthetic blood shot at 80 mm, 120 mm, or 160 mm of mercury (Hg). This is important because the usual arterial pressure of blood is at least 80 mm Hg. A mask that says fluid resistant only has to pass at one of the three pressures. As one can imagine, the only time this will be important is if there is likelihood that there will be splashing of bodily fluids directly on the mask.

The next test for masks is particle filtration efficiency (PFE) that measures the filtration of solid particles at usually 0.1 microns, which is about the size of a small dust particle. This is important if filtration of small particles is important. One can also test for 0.3 micron particle filtration but it is more usual to test for the 0.1 micron standard. See the later paragraph about N95 respirators. Keep in mind that as the measure of filtering small particles improves, less air also can enter a mask for you to breathe. As we increase the number of layers in a mask or the PFE, the less comfortable it will feel, with increased sensation of warmth or air hunger. This is tested as the delta P, or pressure drop, of a mask. If it is less than 2, it is very breathable, and if less than 4 it is moderately breathable, and in most cases should be less than 5. Some masks include a valve that helps with exhalation, but should only be used if the area around the wearer does not need to be sterile and should not be used in areas such as an operating room or procedure field.

Bacterial filtration efficiency is measured as a percentage and should be more than 95-99%. In addition the material should be non-flammable. The American Society for Testing and Materials (ASTM) provides testing methods for each of these tests (ASTM 2100); there are 3 levels of masks based on the above tests, Level 1 through 3. It includes a test for flammability that is standard in all masks to be Class 1 Flammability. Then there are masks that are not assigned a level that either do not submit to the testing or do not meet the criteria. A lack of an assigned level does not imply that it is inferior quality. For example a mask could pass the test for fluid resistance at 80 mm and pass the three other criteria, but if it has a Delta P of 4.4 it could not be given an ASTM Level. Keep in mind that the pressure of arterial blood is 80 to 120 mm. An ASTM Level 1 has fluid resistance to 80 mm Hg, a Delta P Less than 4, and bacterial and particle filtration greater than 95%. An ASTM Level 2 mask has fluid resistance to 120mm Hg, a Delta P less than 5, and bacterial and particle filtration greater than 98%. An ASTM Level 3 mask has fluid resistance to 160 mm Hg, a Delta P less than 5 and bacterial and particle filtration greater than 98%. You can see that the higher the ASTM Level, the greater the protection you receive.

It is readily apparent when shopping for masks that a lot of the above information is not labeled adequately. So how do you choose a mask that will protect you? I see three typical scenarios:

First Scenario. You are travelling on an airplane or you are receiving chemotherapy and you want to avoid respiratory viruses in the air. In this case you only need a Type I or lesser mask that is easily breathable because you will be using the mask for long periods of time. A 2-ply mask will suffice because you do not need any fluid resistance. Keep in mind that none of these masks will completely protect you from small droplet viruses and that some air will get in from around the side of the mask.

Second Scenario. You are changing dressings for a wound with some drainage or you're changing Foley urinary catheters for a loved one. In this case a small amount of fluid resistance will protect you from accidentally splashing bodily fluids into your mouth or nose. A Level I or II fluid resistant mask or any mask labeled fluid resistant will be best.

Third Scenario. You are in an operating room environment where splashing of blood will be brisk arterial flow. You will need a Type II or III mask. Some masks will include a fourth layer with a carbon filter that will filter odors better.

Even more protective than masks are respirators. Some viruses and tuberculosis can travel through the air in smaller particles than bacteria with respirators making claims to protect better from these particles. In order to claim certain protective qualities, a mask must pass not only ASTM measurements but also NIOSH inspections. Respirators include N95 masks which are protective against airborne viruses and tuberculosis, and valved masks, which improve the breathability by providing a second method of air exhalation with an air valve. They also include full-face masks with valves. There are also self-contained respirators that provide an air source within the mask or attached to the mask. These are in general reserved for first responders, hospitals and governmental agencies. So if you do not need a gas mask, these are not for you.

Body coverings are similar to masks in that fluid penetration is important at different pressures, but also time is important here. Gowns can be made from polypropylene or polyethylene. Fluid resistance simply means that it will resist penetration by a small amount (2 ml) of synthetic blood. Some gowns are classified as impervious. These gowns will resist penetration by synthetic blood that remains on the gown for a period of time. This is necessary for operating room environments and situations that require longer duration of wearing while changing dressings that are extensive and soiled. Even more protective are impenetrable materials are used for significant biohazards such as Ebola or plague, etc. Foot coverings are classified according to the same specifications and also usually include non-skid bottoms.

Gloves are made from a variety of materials and thicknesses. They can be made from vinyl or a latex-free rubber material often called Nitrile. Nitrile gloves are usually far more comfortable than vinyl. They can be powder free or with a small amount of powder to help with putting the gloves on. Most gloves are now powder free. Medical grade gloves are made to a higher quality standard. They are measured by penetration of sharp materials, tensile strength, and by fluid penetration. They can also be specified to resist penetration of chemotherapy drugs. Gloves in a box are clean but not sterile. Sterile gloves come in plastic packs of two gloves,

Choosing the correct PPE can be difficult. A lot of research will be needed to determine the level of protection that you require. If you try to think of the bugs you are trying to prevent and how they might bypass your protection, it will be intuitive as to your needs. It is okay to exceed your needs if you do not mind the slight lack of comfort.

Now that you have your PPE, you need to know how to use it. Prior to putting on the PPE you need to wash your hands. If you are using a mask, head covers, or eyewear, put these on now. Then foot covers are put on. If you are double gloving (which is not usually recommended), put the first pair of gloves on now. Put the gown on next, then the first or second pair of gloves. Removing the PPE involves following the directions in the opposite order. If only one set of gloves is used, these come off at the same time as the gown. If two sets of gloves are used, only the first set comes off with the gown. Once the gown and gloves are off, place them in the trash. If they are soiled with a lot of biological fluids, you will need to arrange a method of biohazard disposal. If your mask, head cover, eyewear, or foot covers are soiled, you will need to put on a fresh set of gloves to remove them. Once these are removed and disposed of you will need to wash your hands.

Now you have the tools to protect yourself from whatever may be lurking around the corner. From caring to a loved one's wounds to providing care to someone in an emergency or disaster situation, if you have a safety kit with a few elements from the PPE list above, you will be well prepared. There are some enterprising companies that sell single kits of a gown, gloves and mask that can be placed in your emergency safety kit. Other chapters in this book offer advice on using PPE in specific situations.

Chapter 25

❦

Food Safety

This chapter will be short, because the sheer volume of information will fill an entire book, which will be forthcoming and may already be published by the time you read this book. While outbreaks of infection associated with restaurants and other food establishments occurred long prior to the Jack in the Box and Chipotle events, the widespread reporting of these illnesses would make it seem like these businesses are the only ones with a problem. About once or twice per year, news organizations report on the cases, sensationalizing them as though they are the only cases since the last sensationalized news story. What they do not inform you of, is that every city and state has multiple investigations into food related illnesses every month.

Each city, county, and state has a health department that is tasked with monitoring reports of illnesses that could be communicable in that area. They also have the responsibility to inspect restaurants for cleanliness and food safety practices. These inspections often only uncover the most egregious violations. Some, but not all states require the manager to take a food safety course. Many chain restaurants, even in states without the requirement, have policies in place to make this happen. But what about the Mom and Pop restaurant or the food truck that may not have a true manager besides the owner. These are the places that are more likely to have an outbreak associated with it, relative to the total number of customers.

Likely, all restaurants can and do have small numbers of infections associated with them. Almost all of these mini outbreaks will fly under the radar of the investigators. Illnesses after eating out are so commonplace in our modern society that we often shrug them off as a joke. However, for the more than 100,000 people who are hospitalized and 3,000 who die each year from foodborne infections, they are not a funny joke. Whether at home or in restaurants, we can all make our favorite dining pastime safer for ourselves, friends and family, and our customers.

A few salient points if you know of someone who works in any hospitality industry. First, they need to know that food safety is everyone's responsibility not just the manager. In fact, the dishwasher may have one of the most important jobs. Second, the life they may be protecting may be their own as their exposure to the virus, bacteria, or parasite in the kitchen, dining area, or behind the bar may just as likely make them ill as it will the customer. Lastly, strictly following the rules of food safety is not just for some bureaucrat and is not just to be followed during an inspection. Anyone who has worked in the hospitality knows that during an inspection there are different rules that apply, and as soon as the inspection is over, it is back to the old ways. This is highly unfortunate for you and me because there is a lot of science behind these rules.

Compared to your home kitchen, restaurant kitchens should be treated with a similar but stricter cleaning and sanitizing for food preparation surfaces, cooking surfaces, and dishwashing areas. Use of bleach cleaners are a must for food preparation surfaces. Dishwashing areas need to be kept clean, and the dishwashing water needs to be changed periodically. Insects and rodents should be well controlled. In restaurants there are more than a hundred different safety points to be considered and these can be found in food safety courses and state food safety regulations.

In my subsequent book, I will dissect the restaurant, bar, food truck, and your workplace cafeteria to point out the hidden dangers. The rules will also be dissected to provide a rationale that will be unforgettable for all food service employees allowing them to be able to more easily follow them. For now, if you are a hospitality employee, ask your employer to provide you with the training. Some states have free training available such as New York, which you can access on the internet.

For more information:

https://a816-healthpsi.nyc.gov/dohroot/prjfpc/F2300_Default.aspx

Chapter 26

~

Infections in Dental Settings

Ever since a highly publicized news story in 1990 regarding 6 cases of HIV transmitted by a Florida dentist, we have become more aware of the possibilities of infections during a visit to the dentist. However, I think we still go blindly into the dentist chair and we don't often realize the risk we are about to take. It makes absolute sense that we could contract a disease in this situation. First, we have billions of bacteria in our mouths, highly concentrated in the recesses or cavities of our teeth. Second, the gums and teeth have many blood vessels that create a very bloody scene when the dentist cuts into them. Finally, there can be multiple instances where infections can occur if infection control policies are not strictly adhered to.

The risk of transmission of HIV and Hepatitis B from healthcare workers was well documented in the 1980s and 1990s but since that time there have been very few transmissions. This is likely due to increased vaccinations for Hepatitis B and nearly universal adoption of the use of masks and gloves in the dental office setting. The use of universal precautions (now called standard precautions), which mandates the use of masks and gloves during invasive procedures and while handling contaminated instruments and other materials, has been adopted and adhered to very well since the 1980s. While there have been no cases reported of transmission of Hepatitis C from a dentist, there have been reports of transmission from surgeons performing invasive procedures. Presumably due to the factors listed above it would be exceedingly rare to have a transmission of any of these viruses by a dentist in modern times. However, notwithstanding the above, in 2003 one case was described of transmission of Hepatitis B.

Dental patients and dental health care providers can be exposed to other bacteria and viruses, including cytomegalovirus (CMV), herpes simplex, tuberculosis, staphylococci, and streptococci, and a myriad of other bacteria and viruses that inhabit the mouth. These bacteria and viruses can be transmitted to the patient through direct contact with blood or oral fluids, indirect contact with contaminated objects, or inhalation of microorganisms that can remain suspended in the air for prolonged periods of time. The careful use of standard precautions is instrumental in preventing the transfer of these microorganisms.

The instruments need to be cleaned or sterilized between uses. The CDC classifies instruments and how they are cleaned. Any instruments that come into contact with bone, teeth, gums or non-intact skin need to be sterilized using steam under pressure, dry heat, or chemical vapor. Before sterilizing the instruments need to be cleaned to remove any debris. All other instruments that only come into contact with intact skin such as X-ray heads, blood pressure cuffs, etc. and only need to be cleaned with an intermediate or low level disinfectant. Watch to see what is done with the instruments before and after your visit.

These instruments should be stored in a separate clean room. Temperature and humidity control needs to be in place for this room. In addition, inventory control to assure a sterile instrument's shelf life is not exceeded and instruments sterilized earlier are used first. The packages should be opened in front of the patient and only someone with clean gloves should handle them prior to opening. After opening, only those with appropriate sterile gloves should be handling the instruments and they need to be placed on a clean non-contaminated tray.

The water used to rinse your mouth at the dentist needs to be monitored as it should be as sterile as possible. The use of self-contained water units along with chemical treatment of the water with germicides or the use of inline filters offers the best line of defense against contamination of the dental field. Because bacteria in the patient's mouth can contaminate the instrument that discharges the water, this device needs to be flushed for 30 seconds after each patient.

There have been reports of localized infection or colonization with *Pseudomonas aeruginosa* or *Mycobacterium* species after exposure to water from a dental unit. These are usually diagnosed in immunocompromised individuals, but there is a definite risk if there is not adequate control of these bacteria. Most bacteria in the lines are not a harm to patients, but these two species mentioned above plus potentially Legionella could be spread to patients.

It is highly recommended because of the above concerns that dental healthcare workers be immune or vaccinated against Hepatitis B, Measles, Mumps, Rubella (MMR), varicella (chicken pox), influenza, and Tetanus, Diphtheria, and Pertussis (Tdap). In addition, dental healthcare workers should not come into work if they are ill. The spread of influenza and other illnesses to their patients is very common for all healthcare providers and care to not spread this disease is everyone's job.

So what are the minimum standards that you as a patient can monitor? It would be difficult to monitor most of the above unless you pointedly ask questions about the infection control policies of the office. Hand hygiene with either soap and water or an alcohol-based sanitizer should be used before, during, and after procedures. Watch to see if your providers change their gloves and masks between patients and do they wear protective eyewear? Another thing you can watch for is whether they do flush the devices after they are used on you. There should be impervious barriers (plastic coverings) that cover the parts of instruments that cannot be cleaned and/or you should be able to see the workers diligently cleaning instruments after your time in the chair is finished. Lastly, there should be some form of rinsing of your mouth with an antimicrobial mouth rinse prior to procedures. This mouth rinse can contain either chlorhexidine gluconate or povidone-iodine. If they do not offer it to you, ask for a rinse of chlorhexidine.

You should feel free to ask questions about these practices and any concerns you may have. The dental site OSAP.org has a campaign called "The Safest Dental Visit" that aims to inform patients and dental healthcare providers about what they can do to ensure safe practices. Check it out and arm yourself with information to protect yourself.

More Information:

http://www.cdc.gov/mmwr/preview/mmwrhtml/rr5217a1.htm

Chapter 27

~

Twenty-Five Simple Steps

1.   Obtain a flu shot and pneumonia shot as recommended by your healthcare provider. There are now 2 pneumonia vaccinations and both are recommended for certain individuals.
2.   Prior to elective surgery, wash from head to toe with a chlorhexidine soap daily for 5 days prior to the surgery, as directed by your healthcare provider. There also may be a recommended intranasal ointment to use depending on your facility's policies. Also, get screened for either staph aureus or MRSA colonization with a nasal swab prior to the anesthesia pre-op visit.
3.   Quit smoking prior to a surgical procedure for at least 2 weeks to allow for better blood flow in the wound and therefore better healing and less infections.
4.   Prior to travel to a foreign country, visit a travel medicine clinic and follow the directions for prevention of infections during travel, including vaccinations and malaria prevention. There is information on the CDC's website for travelers.
5.   If you are born between 1945 and 1965, have used intravenous drugs and/or intranasal drugs, or have an unregulated tattoo, you should get tested for Hepatitis C and get treated if necessary. We have cures for Hepatitis C that are less toxic and more effective than in the past.
6.   If you have risk factors for tuberculosis, such as having been exposed to someone with TB in the past, being in jail ever, being homeless ever, working in healthcare, or having emigrated from outside the US, you should be tested with either a PPD skin test

or a blood test using an interferon gamma release assay (IGRA). If positive, almost everyone should be treated, irrespective of whether they received a vaccine against TB.

7. When in the hospital, a nursing facility, or any outpatient health care facility, insist that all workers wash their hands with an alcohol based hand sanitizer each and every time that they enter your room and when they exit your room. Ask for an extra alcohol foam dispenser and place it in a conspicuous place next to you such as on the tray table.

8. If you are sexually active, no matter your age, use condoms. Get checked regularly for STDs including HPV in women with a regular pap smear. Ask for HIV blood or swab tests and tests for syphilis, chlamydia, and gonorrhea.

9. Get regular checks for diabetes especially if you are overweight or over 50. If you have diabetes, maintain regular appointments with a podiatrist and never walk barefoot even around your house. Be careful about walking long distances, especially with improper footwear, and inspect your feet nightly. Treat dry, cracking feet aggressively with antifungal creams or powders.

10. While receiving chemotherapy, do not eat fresh fruits or vegetables unless they are peeled or cooked. In addition, take exquisite care of your port and avoid people who are ill.

11. If you have frequent urinary infections, there may be ways to decrease the number of infections. Cranberry juice and pills may offer some protection and there are some prescription medications such as methenamine or methylene blue that, while not 100% effective, may decrease the number of infections. Someone with 6 infections per year may have only 4. Women may try estrogen creams to thicken the skin near the urethra and this anecdotally may help.

12. While travelling, avoid fresh water for drinking and eating unless bottled. This includes avoidance of foods not cooked and fresh vegetables and fruits that are not peeled or cooked. Salads are out of the question. The rule of thumb is that if there is a possibility that water has touched the part of the food that you eat, either in irrigation or in preparation, you should not consume it. If it is not hot when it touches your lips, do not eat it.

13. If you are hospitalized, bring your own bleach wipes and clean your bed rails, tray table, IV pole, and bathroom upon arrival and daily. Monitor soiling of the bed and insist on cleaning up messes quickly.

14. When swimming and doing water activities that involve dunking the nose below water in freshwater streams, lakes, rivers and ponds, use a nose clip to prevent primary amoebic meningoencephalitis (PAM), which kills more than 8 young people per year in the summertime in the US.

15. Educate yourself and become familiar with Tetanus (Lockjaw) and Pertussis (Whooping Cough) and get vaccinated at least every 10 years with the Tdap vaccination. It could save your life.

16. To prevent pneumonia while in the hospital or rehab/nursing facility utilize a small machine called incentive spirometer 10 times per hour. In addition, when eating or drinking sit straight up in bed, never use a straw, and tilt the chin to the chest when swallowing to avoid aspiration.

17. If you are in a nursing facility during the flu season and a fellow resident contracts influenza, request a preventive dose of oseltamivir to prevent influenza.

18. Use antibiotics judiciously, finish the entire prescription, and never use leftover antibiotics. Eat yogurt or use probiotic pills while on antibiotics if recommended by your doctor.

19. If your children are 12 years of age, obtain the HPV (Human Papillomavirus) vaccine for them and before they head to college obtain both Meningococcal vaccines for them.

20. If you have any issues with wound healing after surgery, immediately seek medical advice from both your surgeon and your primary care physician. Then, immediately contact a wound care center to be seen there as well.

21. If you are pregnant or considering becoming pregnant, read the latest chapter in the CDC's website on prevention of Zika virus at: http://www.cdc.gov/zika/ and become educated on the recent spread of Zika virus.

22. If you have diabetes, monitor your feet nightly to assess for any callouses or wounds. Have your feet assessed regularly by a podiatrist. Do not walk barefoot even inside and try to only use new well-fitted shoes.

23. If you have a Foley catheter or suprapubic catheter, make sure the insertion technique is followed aseptically or sterilely and you need to eliminate dependent loops.

24. At the dentist, monitor the sterile equipment and the water supply. Make sure the equipment appears new and up to date.

25. Always take the recommended duration of your prescription of antibiotics and do not take leftover antibiotics for another infection without consulting your healthcare provider. Prior to taking any antibiotics, discuss with your doctor, the risks and benefits of taking them. Also discuss with your pharmacist any drug interactions or side effects that could be associated with the prescribed antibiotics.

Protect Yourself

∿

About the Author

Dr. Laartz's passion in life is helping people understand how to protect themselves from infection and deal with an infection that has already occurred. The infectious disease doctor is always ready to share an anecdote to help someone understand a disease that may be affecting them or a loved one. He started the series "Protect Yourself" and the company Protect U Guard to help educate individuals on what they need to do to protect themselves from infections.

Dr. Laartz is a board certified infectious diseases specialist in Safety Harbor, Florida with years of experience in infection control at hospitals, nursing facilities, rehab facilities and outpatient clinics. He graduated with his BA and MS degrees from Northwestern University in Evanston, Illinois and his MD degree in 1998 from the University of Iowa in Iowa City, Iowa. He finished his training in Tampa, Florida, where he completed a residency in internal medicine and a fellowship in infectious diseases and tropical medicine at the University of South Florida. He served as chief Infectious Disease Fellow while at the University of South Florida and learned the skills to treat patients with infections. His interest in preventing infections started during this time as he was able to participate in infection prevention rounds at Tampa General Hospital, which he considers one of the great examples of infection control at a teaching hospital.

In Safety Harbor, Florida, he founded and continues to run a successful practice where he has treated patients with almost every infectious disease imaginable. The practice has grown to four physicians and two nurse practitioners. Dr Laartz is on staff at eight local hospitals and runs two outpatient locations. He teaches frequently, holding a teaching appointment as Affiliate Associate Professor of Infectious Diseases and Tropical Medicine at the University of South Florida. Dr Laartz is faculty for two residency programs and teaches for a pharmacy residency and fellowship program. He has served as infection control director and hospital epidemiologist for multiple hospitals. His state of the art clinic in travel medicine offers vaccines, preventive treatment and counseling for travelers. All too often, he has seen diabetic and immunocompromised patients and returning travelers suffer from preventable infections. Dr. Laartz has travelled around the world offering medical assistance wherever needed. He has participated in medical missions to India and has provided care to indigent patients in the Caribbean. For 2 years, while living in the Virgin Islands, he provided education to healthcare providers and patients alike regarding widespread infections such as HIV and tuberculosis.

Through years of practice Dr. Laartz has continued to develop the knowledge to treat some of the most complex infections. Along with this experience comes first hand observation to the many reasons we come down with infections and what predicaments we put ourselves into when we lack common sense. From his medical and travel experience he has learned techniques to prevent infections. In hospitals, he has seen firsthand what works in preventing infections, but also has seen some of the faults in the system patients need to avoid. Not infallible, he has developed infections while travelling, such as one unfortunate episode resulting from eating lobster with a salad at a seaside restaurant in Costa Rica. He is sharing the fruits of this research with the public to help avoid the same infections he has seen day in and day out in the hospital. Many suggestions are so simple that they seem like common sense: however, if common sense was common, we wouldn't need these reminders.

He also performs consulting work for corporations and other organizations to help prevent infections in the workplace and in places where the public congregates, including gyms, restaurants, and churches. Identifying the potential hazards and risks that may lurk at your job, supermarket or your local gym and the best way for these organizations to minimize these risks is no small task. All too often, employers and corporations do not have the guidance necessary. The Occupational Safety and Health

Administration (OSHA) provides some guidance, but, as is sometimes discovered, lessons are learned the hard way. An ounce of prevention is worth a pound of cure any day when it comes to infections.

In order to further empower individuals who wish to avoid infections, he has founded, and is currently creating a company whose vision is to provide quality safety and infection prevention tools directly to the public. He observed that when people need these medical supplies, the cost is prohibitive because they cannot order mass quantities. Protect U Guard, LLC cuts these costs for the average consumers so they can protect themselves better.

In his spare time Dr. Laartz enjoys mountain biking, sailing, boating and scuba diving. Every chance he gets he plays soccer and baseball and travels the globe with his children. Originally from Iowa, he places a great importance on family and his friends. He supports local charities and food markets and enjoys the arts such as opera and Broadway plays. He is extremely passionate about hockey. He is passionate about helping provide access to care for persons with chronic diseases like HIV and helping the public get access to preventive education information. He works tirelessly educating healthcare providers about the simple things they can do to protect their patients. He is penning a book titled "Protect Yourself and Your Patients: Save a Life From Health Care Related Infections", that is geared toward health professionals and how they can understand infection control. Look for it soon.

www.ingramcontent.com/pod-product-compliance
Lightning Source LLC
Chambersburg PA
CBHW060041030426
42334CB00019B/2439